DELMAR'S

Mini Guide

to Pediatric Drugs

George R. Spratto, PhD
Dean Emeritus and Professor
School of Pharmacy
West Virginia University
Morgantown, West Virginia

NOTICE TO THE READER

The monographs in *Delmar's Mini Guide to Pediatric Drugs* is the work of distinguished author George R. Spratto, PhD, Dean Emeritus and Professor of Pharmacology of the School of Pharmacy at West Virginia University, Morgantown, West Virginia.

The publisher and the author do not warrant or guarantee any of the products described herein or perform any independent analysis in connection with any of the product information contained herein. The publisher and the author do not assume and expressly disclaim any obligation to obtain and include information other than that provided by the manufacturer.

The reader is expressly warned to consider and adopt all safety precautions that might be indicated by the activities described herein and to avoid all potential hazards. By following the instructions contained herein, the reader willingly assumes all risks in connection with such instructions.

The publisher and the author make no representations or warranties of any kind, including but not limited to the warranties of fitness for a particular purpose or merchantability nor are any such representations implied with respect to the material set forth herein, and the publisher and the author take no responsibility with respect to such material. The publisher and the author shall not be liable for any special, consequential, or exemplary damages resulting, in whole or in part, from the reader's use of, or reliance upon, this material.

The author and publisher have made a conscientious effort to ensure that the drug information and recommended dosages in this book and companion web site are accurate and in accord with accepted standards at the time of publication. However, pharmacology and therapeutics are rapidly changing sciences, so readers are advised, before administering any drug, to check the package insert provided by the manufacturer for the recommended dose, for any contraindications for administration, and for any added warnings and precautions. This recommendation is especially important for new, infrequently used, or highly toxic drugs.

TABLE OF CONTENTS

PREFACE

Delmar's Mini Guide to Pediatric Drugs consists of approximately 100 drugs that may be prescribed or used in pediatric clients. The cards are intended to be a quick reference source for important information about the drug.

USING THE DRUG CARDS

The following components are described in the order in which they appear on the cards. Please note that the information presented for each drug is not comprehensive; the reader should consult other sources, such as *Delmar 2010 Edition Nurse's Drug Handbook*™, for more complete information.

- **Drug Name:** The generic drug name is the first item in the name block (in color at the beginning of each monograph).
- **Phonetic Pronunciation:** All generic drug names include phonetic pronounciation.
- **Trade Name:** Trade names are identified as OTC (over-the counter, no prescription required) or Rx (prescription).
- ■ **Black Box Warning:** The black box icon indicates that the FDA has issued a boxed warning about potentially dangerous or life-threatening side effects. The actual black box warning is found in the accompanying online companion (OLC), available at http://www.delmarlearning.com/companions.
- **Pregnancy Category:** The FDA pregnancy category (A, B, C, D, or X) assigned to the drug is indicated.
- **Controlled Substance:** If the drug is controlled by the U.S. Federal Controlled Substances Act, the schedule in which the drug is placed (C-II, C-III, C-IV, or C-V) follows the trade name listing.
- **Classification:** The type of drug or the drug class under which the drug is listed is defined.
- **Uses:** Approved therapeutic uses for the drug in the pediatric population are included. Note that the drug may be used for the same or other purposes in other populations of clients.
- **Action/Kinetics:** The action portion describes the proposed mechanism(s) by which a drug achieves its therapeutic effect. Not all mechanisms of action are known, and some are self-evident, as when a hormone is administered as a replacement. The kinetics portion lists critical information, if known, about the rate of drug absorption (including, when known, the percent bioavailable), distribution, time for peak plasma levels or peak effect, minimum effective serum or plasma levels, biological half-life, duration of action, metabolism, and ex-

cretion route(s). Metabolism and excretion may be important for clients with systemic liver disease, kidney disease, or both.

The half-life (**t ½**—the time required for one-half the drug to be excreted or removed from the blood, serum, or plasma) is important in determining how often a drug is to be administered and how long the client is to be assessed for side effects. Therapeutic levels indicate the desired concentration, in serum or plasma, for the drug to exert its beneficial effect and are helpful in predicting the onset of side effects or lack of drug effect.

- **Side Effects:** Listed are the most common undesired or bothersome effects the client may experience while taking a particular drug. In addition, potentially life-threatening side effects are displayed in red italics. Note that the side effects presented are not comprehensive for that particular drug.
- **Dosage:** The dosage form/route of administration and disease state (both in color) for use in the pediatric client are given followed by the dosage for the pediatric client. For ease of reading, shading separates dosages for various uses.

  The listed dosage is to be considered as a general guideline; the exact amount of the drug to be given is determined by the provider. However, one should question orders when dosages differ markedly from the accepted norm. Note that the same or other dosage forms, routes of administration, uses, and dosages may be appropriate for other groups of clients. Appropriate sources should be consulted for this information.
- **Need to Know:** This numbered list provides information on important contraindications, special concerns, drug interactions, and nursing considerations (including administration and client information) for the pediatric client. This list is not intended to be complete; the reader must consult more comprehensive resources for this information.

ACKNOWLEDGMENTS

I would like to extend my thanks and appreciation to the Delmar Cengage Learning team who works so diligently to ensure that the manuscript process flows smoothly and keeps the schedule moving. Team members include Matthew Kane, Director of Learning Solutions; Maureen Rosener, Senior Acquisitions Editor; Beth Williams, Senior Product Manager; Stacey Lamodi, Senior Content Project Manager; Jack Pendleton, Senior Art Director; Mary Colleen Liburdi, Senior Technology Product Manager; and Erin Zeggert, Technology Project Manager.

I also extend greatest appreciation and love to my wife, Lynne, as well as my son Chris and his family (daughter-in-law Mary Alice and grandchildren Patrick Santopietro and Victoria Santopietro) and my son Gregg and his family (daughter-in-law Kim and grandchildren Alexandra and Dominic)—all of whom make the work of this project worthwhile by their unfailing support and encouragement.

George Spratto

Acetaminophen (APAP) **B**
(ah-**SEAT**-ah-**MIN**-oh-fen)

OTC: Drops: Children's Dynafed Jr., Children's Mapap, Infantaire, Infants' Pain Reliever, Liquiprin Drops for Children. **Elixir:** Genapap Children's, Mapap Children's, Silapap Children's, Tylenol Children's. **Oral Liquid/Syrup:** Halenol Children's, Panadol Children's, Silapap Children's, Tempra 2 Syrup. **Oral Solution:** Acetaminophen Drops, Genapap Infants' Drops, Mapap Infant Drops, Panadol Infants' Drops, Silapap Infants, Tempra 1, Tylenol Infants' Drops. **Capsules, Sprinkle:** Feverall Children's, Feverall Junior Strength. **Suppositories:** Children's Feverall, Feverall Suppositories, Infant's Feverall, Junior Strength Feverall. **Tablets, Chewable/Dispersible:** Children's Genapap, Children's Panadol, Children's Tylenol Soft Chews, Tylenol Children's, Tylenol Children's Meltaways. **Tablets:** Tylenol Junior Strength. **Tablets, Oral Disintegrating:** Tylenol Meltaways Jr.

CLASSIFICATION(S): Non-narcotic analgesic

USES: (1) Control of pain due to headache, earache, immunizations, teething, tonsillectomy. (2) To reduce fever in bacterial or viral infections.

ACTION/KINETICS: Decreases fever by (1) a hypothalamic effect leading to sweating and vasodilation and (2) inhibits the effect of pyrogens on the hypothalamic heat-regulating centers. May cause analgesia by inhibiting CNS prostaglandin synthesis. Does not cause any anticoagulant effect or ulceration of the GI tract. Antipyretic and analgesic effects are comparable to those of aspirin. **Peak plasma levels:** 30–120 min. **$t\frac{1}{2}$:** 45 min–3 hr. **Therapeutic serum levels** (analgesia): 5–20 mcg/mL. Metabolized in the liver and excreted in the urine as glucuronide and sulfate conjugates.

SIDE EFFECTS: Few when taken in usual therapeutic doses. GI upset in some.

DOSAGE: Caplets; Capsules; Capsules, Sprinkle; Elixir; Gelcaps; Oral Liquid/Syrup; Oral Solution; Syrup; Tablets; Tablets, Chewable; Tablets, Dispersible

Analgesic, antipyretic.

Children: Doses given 4–5 times per day. **Up to 3 months:** 40 mg/dose; **4–11 months:** 80 mg/dose; **1–2 years:** 120 mg/dose; **2–3 years:** 160 mg/dose; **4–5 years:** 240 mg/dose; **6–8 years:** 320 mg/dose; **9–10 years:** 400 mg/dose; **11 years:** 480 mg/dose; **12–14 years:** 640 mg/dose; **over 14 years:** 650 mg/dose. *Alternative children dose:* 10–15 mg/kg q 4 hr.

DOSAGE: Suppositories

Analgesic, antipyretic.

Children, 3–11 months: 80 mg q 6 hr; **1–3 years:** 80 mg q 4 hr; **3–6 years:** 120–125 mg q 4–6 hr, with no more than 720 mg in 24 hr; **6–12 years:** 325 mg q 4–6 hr with no more than 2.6 grams in 24 hr. Given as needed while symptoms persist.

DOSAGE: Tablets, Extended-Release

Children, over 12 years: 1,300 mg (2 tablets) q 8 hr, up to 6 tablets/day.

DOSAGE: Tablets, Oral Disintegrating

Analgesic, antipyretic.

Children, 6–8 years: 320 mg (2 tablets) q 4 hr, up to 10 per day; **9–10 years:** 400 mg (2½ tablets) q 4 hr, up to 12½ tablets per day; **11 years:** 480 mg (3 tablets) q 4 hr, up to 15 tablets per day; **12 years:** 640 mg (4 tablets) q 4 hr, up to 20 tablets per day.

NEED TO KNOW

1. Toxicity, including serious liver damage (hepatocyte necrosis) and apoptosis, may occur with doses not far beyond labeled dosing, especially when using high doses and when taking more than one product containing acetaminophen.
2. Do not exceed 75 mg/kg/day in children.

3. Do not take for more than 5 days for pain in children or more than 3 days for fever in children without consulting provider.
4. Bubble gum flavored OTC pediatric products (liquid and chewable tablets) are available to treat fever and/or pain.
5. Do not combine products containing acetaminophen, many of which are OTC. Read labels on all OTC products consumed.
6. Review with parents the difference between concentrated dropper dose formulation and teaspoon dose formulation.

Albuterol (Salbutamol) C

(al-**BYOU**-ter-ohl)

Rx: AccuNeb, ProAir HFA, Proventil, Proventil HFA, Ventolin, Ventolin HFA, VoSpire ER.

CLASSIFICATION(S): Sympathomimetic

USES: Inhalation: (1) Prophylaxis and relief of bronchospasm in reversible obstructive airway disease. (2) Acute attacks of bronchospasm (inhalation solution). (3) Prophylaxis of exercise-induced bronchospasm. **Syrup:** Relief of bronchospasm in children 2 years and older with reversible obstructive airway disease. **Tablets and Extended-Release Tablets:** Relief of bronchospasm in children 6 years and older with reversible obstructive airway disease.

ACTION/KINETICS: Stimulates beta-2 receptors of the bronchi, leading to bronchodilation. **Onset, PO:** 15–30 min; **inhalation,** within 5 min. **Peak effect, PO:** 2–3 hr; **inhalation,** 60–90 min (after 2 inhalations). **Duration, PO:** 4–8 hr (up to 12 hr for extended-release); **inhalation,** 3–6 hr. Metabolites and unchanged drug excreted in urine and feces.

SIDE EFFECTS: Headache, N&V, palpitations/tachycardia, tremor, bronchospasm. *ANGIOEDEMA, BRONCHOSPASM.*

DOSAGE: Inhalation Aerosol

Bronchodilation.

Children, over 4 years (12 and over for Proventil): 180 mcg (2 inhalations) q 4–6 hr. In some clients 1 inhalation (90 mcg) q 4 hr may be sufficient. **Maintenance (Proventil only):** 180 mcg (2 inhalations) 4 times per day.

Prophylaxis of exercise-induced bronchospasm.

Children, over 4 years (12 and over for Proventil): 180 mcg (2 inhalations) 15 min before exercise.

DOSAGE: Inhalation Solution

Bronchodilation.

Children, over 12 years: 2.5 mg 3–4 times per day by nebulization (dilute 0.5 mL of the 0.5% solution with 2.5 mL sterile NSS and deliver over 5–15 min); **2–12 years (15 kg or over), initial:** 2.5 mg (1 UD vial) 3–4 times per day by nebulization. **Children, weighing less than 15 kg who require less than the 2.5 mg dose (i.e., less than a full UD vial):** Use the 0.5% inhalation solution. Give over about 5–15 min.

DOSAGE: Accuneb

Relief and prophylaxis of bronchospasms.

Initial, children 2–12 years: 1.25 mg or 0.63 mg given 3–4 times per day, as needed, by nebulization. Do not give more frequently. Administer over about 5–15 min.

DOSAGE: Syrup

Bronchodilation.

Children, over 6–12 years, initial: 2 mg (5 mL) 3–4 times per day; **then,** increase as necessary to a maximum of 24 mg/day in divided doses. **2–6 years, initial:** 0.1 mg/kg 3 times per day, not to exceed 2 mg (5 mL) 3 times per day; **then,** increase as necessary up to 0.2 mg/kg 3 times per day, not to exceed 4 mg (10 mL) 3 times per day.

DOSAGE: Tablets

Bronchodilation.

Children, over 12 years, initial: 2 or 4 mg 3–4 times per day; **then,** increase dose as needed up to a maximum of 8 mg 4 times per day, as tolerated. Increase dose gradually, if needed, to a maximum of 8 mg 3–4 times per day, not to exceed 32 mg/day in children over 12 years. **6–12 years, usual, initial:** 2 mg 3–4 times per day; **then,** if necessary, increase the dose in a stepwise fashion to a maximum of 24 mg/day in divided doses.

DOSAGE: Vospire ER Tablets

Bronchodilation.

Children, over 12 years: 8 mg q 12 hr; in some clients, 4 mg q 12 hr may be sufficient initially and then increased to 8 mg q 12 hr, depending on the response. The dose can be increased stepwise and cautiously (under provider supervision) to a maximum of 32 mg/day in divided doses q 12 hr. **6–12 years:** 4 mg q 12 hr. The dose can be increased stepwise and cautiously (under provider supervision) to a maximum of 24 mg/day in divided doses q 12 hr.

NEED TO KNOW

1. The aerosol and inhalation powder are indicated for children 4 years and older (12 years and older for Proventil); the solution for inhalation is indicated for children 2 years and older.
2. When given by nebulization, use either a face mask or mouthpiece. Use compressed air or oxygen with a gas flow of 6–10 L/min; a single treatment lasts from 5 to 15 min.
3. Contents of the MDI container are under pressure. Do not store near heat or open flames and do not puncture the container.
4. AccuNeb, either 0.63 mg/3 mL or 1.25 mg/3 mL is intended for relief of bronchospasm in children 2–12 years of age with asthma.
5. A spacer used with the MDI may enhance drug dispersion. Always thoroughly rinse mouth and equipment with water following each use to prevent oral fungal infections.
6. Use caution, may cause dizziness/drowsiness.

Amoxicillin (Amoxycillin) **B**

(ah-mox-ih-**SILL**-in)

Rx: Amoxil, Amoxil Pediatric Drops, DisperMox, Polymox, Trimox.

CLASSIFICATION(S): Antibiotic, penicillin

USES:

(1) Ear, nose, and throat infections due to *Streptococcus* species (α– and β–lactamase-negative only), *S. pneumoniae, Staphylococcus* species, or *Haemophilus influenzae.* (2) GU infections due to *Escherichia coli, Proteus mirabilis,* or *Enterococcus faecalis.* (3) Skin and skin structure infections due to *Streptococcus* species (α– and β–hemolytic strains only), *Staphylococcus* species, or *E. coli.* (4) Lower respiratory tract infections due to *Streptococcus* species (α– and β–hemolytic strains only), *S. pneumoniae, Staphylococcus* species, or *H. haemophilus.* (5) Acute uncomplicated (anogenital and urethral) gonococcal infections due to *Neisseria gonorrhoeae.*

ACTION/KINETICS: Binds to penicillin-binding proteins (PBP-1 and PBP-3) in the cytoplasmic membranes of bacteria, thus inhibiting cell wall synthesis. Cell division and growth are inhibited. **Peak serum levels, PO:** 4–11 mcg/mL after 1–2 hr. **t½:** 60 min. Mostly excreted unchanged in urine.

SIDE EFFECTS: Hypersensitivity, N&V, gastritis, stomatitis.

DOSAGE: Capsules; Oral Suspension; Tablets; Tablets, Chewable

Susceptible infections of ear, nose, throat, GU tract, skin and soft tissues. Mild to moderate infections.

Children, 40 kg and over: 500 mg q 8 hr or 500 mg q 12 hr; **3 months and older and less than 40 kg:** 20 mg/kg/day in divided doses q 8 hr or 25 mg/kg/day in divided doses q 12 hr.

Severe infections.

Children, 40 kg and over: 875 mg q 12 hr or 500 mg q 8 hr; **3 months and over and less than 40 kg:** 45 mg/kg/day in divided doses q 12 hr or 40 mg/kg/day in divided doses q 8 hr. For children, do not exceed the maximum adult dose.

Infections of the lower respiratory tract.

Children, 40 kg and over: 500 mg q 8 hr or 875 mg q 12 hr; **3 months and older and under 40 kg:** 40 mg/kg/day in divided doses q 8 hr or 45 mg/kg/day in divided doses q 12 hr.

Prophylaxis of bacterial endocarditis: dental, oral, respiratory tract, or esophageal; moderate-risk clients undergoing GU/GI procedures.

Children: 50 mg/kg.

Gonococcal infections, uncomplicated urethral, endocervical, or rectal infections.

Children, over 2 years (prepubertal): 50 mg/kg amoxicillin combined with 25 mg/kg probenecid as a single dose.

Anthrax (postexposure prophylaxis following confirmed or suspected exposure to Bacillus anthracis*).*

Children, less than 9 years: 80 mg/kg/day PO divided into 2–3 doses. Continue prophylaxis until exposure has been excluded. If exposure is confirmed and vaccine is available, continue prophylaxis for 4 weeks and until 3 doses of vaccine have been given or for 30–60 days if vaccine is unavailable.

NEED TO KNOW

1. Child's dose should not exceed maximum adult dose.
2. For school-age child space evenly over 24-hr period; give before school, upon arrival home, at bedtime.
3. Chewable tablets available for children; may be taken with food.
4. Place pediatric drops directly on child's tongue to swallow. May add drops to formula, milk, fruit juice, water, ginger ale, or cold drinks; must be taken immediately and consumed completely.
5. Report unusual symptoms, i.e., ↑ bruising/bleeding, sore throat, rash, diarrhea, worsening of symptoms, or lack of response.

Amoxicillin and Potassium clavulanate **B**

(ah-mox-ih-**SILL**-in, poh-**TASS**-ee-um klav-you-**LAN**-ayt)

Rx: Amoclan, Augmentin, Augmentin ES-600, Augmentin XR.

CLASSIFICATION(S): Antibiotic, penicillin

USES: Augmentin. For beta-lactamase-producing strains of the following organisms: (1) Lower respiratory tract infections, otitis media, and sinusitis caused by *Haemophilus influenzae* and *Moraxella catarrhalis.* (2) Skin and skin structure infections caused by *Staphylococcus aureus, Escherichia coli,* and *Klebsiella.* (3) UTI caused by *E. coli, Klebsiella* species, and *Enterobacter.* **Augmentin ES-600.** Recurrent or persistent acute otitis media in pediatric clients due to *Streptococcus pneumoniae* (penicillin MICs less than or equal to 2 mcg/mL), *H. influenzae* (including β-lactamase-producing strains), or *M. catarrhalis* (including β-lactamase-producing strains) characterized by the following risk factors: Antibiotic exposure for acute otitis media within the preceding 3 months and **either** 2 years or younger or daycare attendance. Do not use Augmentin ES-600 to treat acute otitis media due to *S. pneumoniae* with penicillin MIC at least 4 mcg/mL.

ACTION/KINETICS: Potassium clavulanate inactivates lactamase enzymes, which are responsible for resistance to penicillins.

SIDE EFFECTS: Hypersensitivity, N&V, gastritis, stomatitis.

DOSAGE: Oral Suspension; Tablets; Tablets, Chewable

AUGMENTIN

Susceptible infections.

Children, over 40 kg: One 500-mg tablet q 12 hr or one 250-mg tablet q 8 hr; **less than 3 months old:** 30 mg/kg/day amoxicillin in divided doses q 12 hr. Use of the 125-mg/5 mL suspension is recommended. **Over 3 months old:** 200 mg/5 mL or 400 mg/5 mL q 12 hr. Or, 125 mg/5 mL or 250 mg/5 mL q 8 hr.

Recurrent or persistent acute otitis media, sinusitis, lower respiratory tract infections.

Children, 3 months and older: 45 mg/kg/day of amoxicillin in divided doses q 12 hr or 40 mg/kg/day amoxicillin in divided doses q 8 hr. For less severe infections, use 25 mg/kg/day in divided doses q 12 hr or 20 mg/kg/day in divided doses q 8 hr.

DOSAGE: Oral Suspension AUGMENTIN ES-600

Recurrent or persistent acute otitis media in children.

Children, 3 months and older: 90 mg/kg/day amoxicillin in divided doses q 12 hr for 10 days. Experience is not available for pediatric clients weighing more than 40 kg.

NEED TO KNOW

1. Both '250' and '500' tablets contain 125 mg clavulanic acid; therefore, two '250' tablets are not the same as one '500' tablet. The 250-mg tablet and the 250-mg chewable tablet do not contain the same amount of potassium clavulanate and are thus not interchangeable. The 250-mg tablet should not be used until children are over 40 kg.
2. Pediatric formulations are available in fruit flavors for oral suspension and chewable tablets. These formulations allow twice-daily dosing; more convenient than three-times daily dosing; and incidence of diarrhea is significantly reduced.
3. The 200- and 400-mg suspensions and chewable tablets contain aspartame; do not use with phenylketonuria.
4. May take without regard for meals; absorption of potassium clavulanate enhanced if taken just before a meal. To lessen stomach upset, take with food.
5. Do not chew or crush; swallow tablets whole. Consume fluids to ensure adequate hydration.
6. Report side effects, i.e., rash, persistent diarrhea, lack of response, worsening of symptoms after 48–72 hr.
7. Refrigerate reconstituted suspension; discard after 10 days.

Amphetamine mixtures

(am-**FET**-ah-meen) **C**

Rx: Adderall XR, Adderall, Amphetamine Salt Combo, **C-II.**

CLASSIFICATION(S): CNS stimulant

USES: (1) Attention deficit/hyperactivity disorder (ADHD) in children over 3 years, along with other remedial approaches.
(2) Narcolepsy in children over 6 years.

ACTION/KINETICS: Thought to act on the cerebral cortex and reticular activating system by releasing norepinephrine from central adrenergic neurons. Completely absorbed in 3 hr. **Peak effects:** 2–3 hr. **Duration:** 4–24 hr. **Therapeutic blood levels:** 5–10 mcg/dL. **$t^{1/2}$, if urine pH is 5.6 or less:** 7– 8 hr; **$t^{1/2}$, if urine pH is alkaline:** 18.6–33.6 hr.

SIDE EFFECTS: Decreased appetite, upset stomach, insomnia, increased anxiety, irritability.

DOSAGE: Capsules, Extended-Release; Tablets

Attention deficit/hyperactivity disorders.

Children, 3–5 years, initial: 2.5 mg/day; increase by 2.5 mg/day at weekly intervals until optimum dose is achieved (usual range 0.1–0.5 mg/kg/dose each morning); **6 years and older, initial:** 5 mg 1–2 times per day; increase in increments of 5 mg/day at weekly intervals until optimum dose is achieved (only rarely will doses exceed a total of 40 mg/day). For the extended-release capsules, start with 10 mg once daily in the morning; increase in increments of 10 mg/day at weekly intervals, up to a maximum of 30 mg/day.

Narcolepsy.

Children, over 12 years, initial: 10 mg/day; increase in increments of 10 mg/day at weekly intervals until optimum dosage is achieved. **6–12 years, initial:** 5 mg/day; increase in increments of 5 mg/day until optimum dosage is achieved. For all ages, use immediate-release products. Give the first dose on awakening with additional 1–2 doses at intervals of 4–6 hr.

NEED TO KNOW

1. Do not use in children less than 3 years for attention deficit disorders, in children less than 6 years of age for narcolepsy, or in children with a structural cardiac abnormality due to the possibility of sudden death. Do not use as an appetite suppressant.
2. Extended-release amphetamine has not been studied in children less than 6 years.
3. Take extended-release capsules whole or sprinkle contents on applesauce. If applesauce is used, take immediately (do not store). Do not chew applesauce sprinkled with amphetamine beads.
4. The correct dose must be given at the right time; never give doses more than 2 hours late, unless told otherwise by the provider. Never double doses. It is safer for a child to skip a dose than inadvertantly be given two doses.
5. Take with water; do not take with milk, juice, or antacids.
6. Children receiving amphetamines may have growth retarded. Drug should periodically be discontinued (i.e., during the summer) by provider to allow growth to proceed normally and to evaluate the need for continued drug therapy.

Ampicillin oral

(am-pih-**SILL**-in) **B**

Rx: Principen.

Ampicillin sodium, parenteral

Rx: Ampicillin sodium.

CLASSIFICATION(S): Antibiotic, penicillin

USES: (1) Respiratory tract infections. (2) GI infections. (3) GU infections. (4) Use of the injection only for bacterial meningitis due to *Neisseria meningitides*, *E. coli*, *Listeria monocytogenes*, and Group

B streptococci. Addition of an aminoglycoside may enhance effectiveness against gram-negative bacteria. (5) Use of the injection only for septicemia and endocarditis due to *Streptococcus* species, penicillin G susceptible staphylococci, enterococci, *E. coli, P. mirabilis,* and *Salmonella.* Addition of an aminoglycoside may enhance effectiveness when treating streptococcal endocarditis.

ACTION/KINETICS: Synthetic, broad-spectrum antibiotic suitable for gram-negative bacteria. Acid resistant, destroyed by penicillinase. Absorbed more slowly than other penicillins. **Peak serum levels; PO:** 1.8–2.9 mcg/mL after 2 hr; **IM:** 4.5–7 mcg/mL. **$t_{1/2}$:** 80 min–range 50–110 min. Partially inactivated in liver; 25–85% excreted unchanged in urine.

SIDE EFFECTS: Hypersensitivity, N&V, gastritis, stomatitis.

DOSAGE: Ampicillin Oral: Capsules, Oral Suspension; Ampicillin Sodium: IM, IV

Respiratory tract and soft tissue infections.

PO: Children, 20 kg or more: 250 mg q 6 hr; **less than 20 kg:** 50 mg/kg/day in equally divided doses q 6–8 hr. **IV, IM: 40 kg or more:** 250–500 mg q 6 hr; **less than 40 kg:** 25–50 mg/kg/day in equally divided doses q 6–8 hr.

Bacterial meningitis.

Children: 150–200 mg/kg/day in divided doses q 3 to 4 hr. Initially give IV drip, followed by IM q 3 to 4 hr.

Bacterial endocarditis prophylaxis (dental, oral, or upper respiratory tract procedures).

Children, IM, IV: 50 mg/kg, 30 min prior to procedure. **Clients at high risk: Children, IM, IV:** Ampicillin, 50 mg/kg, plus gentamicin, 1.5 mg/kg, 30 min prior to procedure followed in 6 hr by ampicillin, 25 mg/kg IM or IV, or amoxicillin, 25 mg/kg PO.

Septicemia.

Children: 150–200 mg/kg/day, IV for first 3 days, then IM q 3–4 hr.

GI and GU infections, other than N. gonorrhoeae.

Children, more than 20 kg: 500 mg PO q 6 hr. Use larger doses, if needed, for severe or chronic infections. **Less than 20 kg:** 100 mg/kg/day q 6 hr.

N. gonorrhoeae *infections.*

Children, over 40 kg: 500 mg IV or IM q 6 hr. **Less than 40 kg:** 50 mg/kg/day IV or IM in equally divided doses q 6 to 8 hr.

NEED TO KNOW

1. After reconstitution for IM or direct IV administration, solution **must be used within the hour.**
2. Once reconstituted, give IV slowly over at least 10–15 min.
3. Note history of sensitivity/reactions to this or related drugs.
4. Take 1 hr before or 2 hr after meals; food may interfere with absorption.
5. Take for prescribed number of days even if symptoms subside.
6. Ampicillin chewable tablets should not be swallowed whole.
7. Report any 'ampicillin rashes'; a dull, red, itchy, flat, or raised rash occurs more often with this drug than with other penicillins.

Ampicillin sodium/Sulbactam sodium

(am-pih-**SILL**-in, sull-**BACK**-tam)

Rx: Unasyn.

B

CLASSIFICATION(S): Antibiotic, penicillin

USES: (1) Skin and skin structure infections caused by *Staphylococcus aureus, Escherichia coli, Klebsiella* species (including *K. pneumoniae*), *Proteus mirabilis, Bacteroides fragilis, Enterobacter* species, and *Acinetobacter calcoaceticus.* (2) Intra-abdominal infections caused by *E. coli, Klebsiella* species (including *K. pneumoniae*), *Bacteroides* (including *B. fragilis*), and *Enterobacter.*

ACTION/KINETICS: Sulbactam is present in this product because it irreversibly inhibits beta-lactamases, thus ensuring activity of ampicillin against beta-lactamase-producing microorganisms. **Peak serum levels, after IV infusion:** 15 min. **$t^{1/2}$, both drugs:** about 1 hr. From 75–85% of both drugs are excreted unchanged in the urine within 8 hr after administration.

SIDE EFFECTS: Hypersensitivity, N&V, gastritis, stomatitis.

DOSAGE: IM; IV

All infections.

Children, over 40 kg: Use adult doses; total sulbactam dose should not exceed 4 grams/day; **1 year and older but less than 40 kg:** 300 mg/kg/day (200 mg ampicillin/100 mg sulbactam) in divided doses q 6 hr.

NEED TO KNOW

1. Safety and efficacy in children 1 year of age and older have not been established for intra-abdominal infections or for IM administration.
2. Must use solutions for IM administration **within 1 hr** of preparation.
3. IM injections are extremely painful; expect some discomfort. Report if S&S worsen, diarrhea, vaginal itching occurs, or symptoms do not improve.
4. Report any adverse effects including skin rash; if accompanied by fatigue, sore throat, and enlarged spleen and lymph nodes, a heterophil antibody test may be ordered to rule out mononucleosis.

Aspirin (Acetylsalicylic acid, ASA) (ah-**SEE**-till-sal-ih-**SILL**-ick **AH**-sid) ■ C

OTC: Gum Tablets: Aspergum. **Caplets/Tablets:** Bayer Buffered Aspirin, Genuine Bayer Aspirin Caplets and Tablets. **Tablets, Chewable:** Bayer Children's Aspirin. **Tablets, Coated:** Ascriptin, Bufferin. **Tablets, Effervescent:** Alka-Seltzer with Aspirin (Flavored).

CLASSIFICATION(S): Nonsteroidal anti-inflammatory, analgesic, antipyretic

USES: Analgesic: (1) Pain from integumentary structures, myalgias, neuralgias, arthralgias, headache, and similar types of pain. (2) May be effective in less severe postoperative and postpartum pain; pain secondary to trauma and cancer. **Antipyretic, anti-inflammatory:** SLE, acute rheumatic fever, arthritis, and many other conditions.

ACTION/KINETICS: The antipyretic effect is due to an action on the hypothalamus, resulting in heat loss by vasodilation of peripheral blood vessels and promoting sweating. The anti-inflammatory effects are probably mediated through inhibition of cyclo-oxygenase, which results in a decrease in prostaglandin (implicated in the inflammatory response) synthesis and other mediators of the pain response. Aspirin also produces inhibition of platelet aggregation. Rapidly absorbed after PO administration. Is hydrolyzed to the active salicylic acid. Salicylic acid and metabolites are excreted by the kidney. The addition of antacids (buffered aspirin) may decrease GI irritation and increase the dissolution and absorption of such products.

SIDE EFFECTS: Dyspepsia, nausea, epigastric discomfort. The toxic effects of the salicylates are dose-related. *MASSIVE GI BLEEDING, POTENTIATION OF PEPTIC ULCER, BRONCHOSPASM, ASTHMA-LIKE SYMPTOMS, ANAPHYLAXIS.*

DOSAGE: Gum; Suppositories; Tablets, Chewable

Analgesic, antipyretic.

Children: 65 mg/kg/day (alternate dose: 1.5 grams/m^2/day) in divided doses q 4–6 hr, not to exceed 3.6 grams/day. The following dosage regimen can be used: **Children, 2–3 years:** 162 mg q 4 hr as needed; **4–5 years:** 243 mg q 4 hr as needed; **6–8 years:** 320–325 mg q 4 hr as needed; **9–10 years:** 405 mg q 4 hr as needed; **11 years:** 486 mg q 4 hr as needed; **12–14 years:** 648 mg q 4 hr.

Acute rheumatic fever.

Children, initial: 100 mg/kg/day (3 grams/m^2/day) for 2 weeks; **then,** decrease to 75 mg/kg/day for 4–6 weeks.

Juvenile rheumatoid arthritis.

60–110 mg/kg/day (alternate dose: 3 grams/m^2/day in divided doses q 6–8 hr. When ititiating therapy at 60 mg/kg/day, dose may be increased by 20 mg/kg/day after 5–7 days and by 10 mg/kg/day after another 5–7 days.

NEED TO KNOW

1. Do not use in children or teenagers with chickenpox or flu symptoms due to the possibility of Reye's syndrome, a rare but serious illness.
2. Asthma caused by hypersensitivity reaction to salicylates may be refractory to epinephrine, so antihistamines should also be available for parenteral and PO use.
3. Salicylates should be administered to children only upon specific medical order related to risk of Reye's syndrome.
4. If child refuses medication or vomits it, consider suppositories or acetaminophen.
5. Dehydrated children who have a fever are especially susceptible to aspirin intoxication from even small doses.

Atomoxetine HCl
(**AT**-oh-mox-eh-teen)
Rx: Strattera.

CLASSIFICATION(S): Drug for attention-deficit/hyperactivity disorder

USES: Attention-deficit/hyperactivity disorder (ADHD) as categorized by DSM-IV-TR.

ACTION/KINETICS: Thought to be related to selective inhibition of presynaptic norepinephrine transport, thus increasing levels of norepinephrine in nerve synapses. Rapidly absorbed after PO use. High fat meals decrease the rate of absorption. **Maximum plasma levels:** 1–2 hr. **t½:** About 5 hr. **Plasma protein binding:** About 98%.

SIDE EFFECTS: Dyspepsia, N&V, fatigue, decreased appetite, dizziness, mood swings.

DOSAGE: Capsules

ADHD.

Children, over 70 kg, initial: Total daily dose of 40 mg. May increase after a minimum of 3 days to a target total daily dose of about 80 mg given either as a single dose in the a.m. or as evenly divided doses in the morning and late afternoon/early evening. After 2–4 weeks, dose may be increased to a maximum of 100 mg in those who have not achieved an optimal response. **Children, up to 70 kg, initial:** Total daily dose of about 0.5 mg/kg. May be increased after a minimum of 3 days to a target total daily dose of about 1.2 mg/kg given either as a single dose in the a.m. or as evenly divided doses in the morning and late afternoon/early evening. Do not exceed a maximum daily dose of 1.4 mg/kg or 100 mg, whichever is less.

NEED TO KNOW

1. Safety and efficacy have not been determined in children younger than 6 years of age.

2. Take with or without food.
3. Periodically evaluate the long-term usefulness for each client.
4. For children and adolescents up to 70 kg who have been given fluoxetine, quinidine, or paroxetine, initiate dosage at 0.5 mg/kg/day and only increase to the usual target dose of 1.2 mg/kg/day if symptoms fail to improve after 4 weeks and initial dose is well tolerated.

Azithromycin
(ah-**zith**-roh-**MY**-sin) **B**

Rx: AzaSite Ophthalmic Solution, Zithromax, Zmax.

CLASSIFICATION(S): Antibiotic, macrolide

USES: **Children, Oral:** (1) Acute otitis media due to *H. influenzae, M. catarrhalis,* or *S. pneumoniae* in children over 6 months of age. (2) Acute bacterial sinusitis in children 6 months and older due to *H. influenzae, M. catarrhalis*, or *S. pneumoniae*. (3) CAP due to *C. pneumoniae, H. influenzae, M. pneumoniae,* or *S. pneumoniae* in children over 6 months of age who can take PO therapy.
(4) Pharyngitis/tonsillitis due to *S. pyogenes* in children over 2 years who cannot use first-line therapy. Penicillin IM is the usual drug of choice to treat *S. pyogenes* infections and for prophylaxis of rheumatic fever.

ACTION/KINETICS: Acts by binding to the P site of the 50S ribosomal subunit and may inhibit RNA-dependent protein synthesis by stimulating the dissociation of peptidyl t-RNA from ribosomes. Rapidly absorbed and distributed widely throughout the body. Food increases the absorption of azithromycin. Mainly excreted unchanged through the bile with a small amount being excreted through the kidneys.

SIDE EFFECTS: Abdominal pain/discomfort, N&V, anorexia, diarrhea/loose stools, injection site reactions (local inflammation, pain), pruritis, rash, vaginitis.

DOSAGE: Oral Suspension

Otitis media or CAP.

Children, 6 months and older weighing at least 5 kg, 5-day regimen: 10 mg/kg as a single dose (not to exceed 500 mg) on day 1, followed by 5 mg/kg (not to exceed 250 mg/day) on days 2 through 5. **Children, 6 months and older weighing at least 5 kg, 3-day regimen for otitis media:** 10 mg/kg/day. **Children, 6 months and older weighing at least 5 kg, 1-day regimen for otitis media:** 30 mg/kg as a single dose.

Pharyngitis/tonsillitis.

Children: 12 mg/kg once daily for 5 days, not to exceed 500 mg/day.

Chlamydial infections caused by C. trachomatis.

Children, 45 kg or more, and less than 8 years; or over 8 years: 1 gram given as a single dose.

Acute bacterial sinusitis.

Children, 6 months and older: 10 mg/kg once daily for 3 days.

NEED TO KNOW

1. Safety and efficacy for acute otitis media have not been determined in children less than 6 months of age or for pharyngitis/tonsillitis in children less than 2 years.
2. Tablets and oral suspension can be taken with or without food; however, there is increased tolerability when tablets are taken with food (can be taken with milk).
3. Notify provider if N&V or diarrhea is excessive or debilitating.
4. Avoid sun exposure and use protection when outside.

Benzonatate

(ben-**ZOH**-nah-tayt)

Rx: Tessalon Perles.

C

CLASSIFICATION(S): Antitussive, nonnarcotic

USES: Symptomatic relief of cough.

ACTION/KINETICS: Anesthetizes stretch receptors in respiratory passages, lungs, and pleura reducing their activity and decreasing the cough reflex at its source. **Onset:** 15–20 min. **Duration:** 3–8 hr.

SIDE EFFECTS: GI upset, nausea, constipation, drowsiness, dizziness, nasal congestion, headache. *BRONCHOSPASM, LARYNGOSPASM, CV COLLAPSE, CHOKING*.

DOSAGE: Capsules (Perles)

Antitussive.

Children, over 10 years: 100–200 mg 3 times per day, up to a maximum of 600 mg/day.

NEED TO KNOW

1. Safety and efficacy have not been determined in children less than 10 years.
2. Take only as directed and with plenty of fluids. Swallow perles whole without chewing or crushing to avoid local anesthetic effect on oral mucosa and to prevent choking.
3. Report if symptoms intensify or do not improve after 5 days. Avoid all triggers/irritants such as dust, smoke, strong odors, and fumes. Keep all follow up appointments.

Budesonide

(byou-**DES**-oh-nyd)

B

Rx: Capsules: Entocort EC. **Inhalation**: Pulmicort Flexhaler, Pulmicort Respules, Pulmicort Turbuhaler. **Intranasal**: Rhinocort Aqua.

CLASSIFICATION(S): Glucocorticoid

USES: (1) Pulmicort Flexhaler: Prophylaxis and maintenance treatment of asthma in children 6 years and older, including those requiring PO corticosteroid therapy for asthma. (2) **Pulmicort Respules:** Prophylaxis and maintenance treatment of asthma in children and infants 6 months to 8 years. (3) **Pulmicort Turbuhaler:** Maintenance treatment of asthma as prophylaxis in children 6 years and older; also for those requiring oral corticosteroid therapy for asthma. (4) **Rhinocort Aqua:** Treat symptoms of seasonal or perennial allergic rhinitis in children 6 years and older.

ACTION/KINETICS: Exerts a direct local anti-inflammatory effect with minimal systemic effects when used intranasally. **Onset, nasal spray:** 10 hr. **t½:** 2–3 hr. Excreted through both urine and feces.

SIDE EFFECTS: Inhalation Powder: Headache, URTI, flu-like symptoms, sinusitis, pharyngitis, back pain/pain, bronchospasm, cough, epistaxis. **Inhalation Suspension:** URTI, rhinitis, nasal congestion, otitis media/ear infection, epistaxis. *IMMEDIATE AND DELAYED HYPERSENSITIVITY REACTIONS TO ALL PRODUCTS.*

DOSAGE: Pulmicort Respules

Prophylaxis and maintenance treatment of asthma.

Children, 12 months to 8 years: If previous therapy was bronchodilators alone: 0.5 mg total daily dose given either once or twice daily in divided doses (maximum daily dose: 0.5 mg). If previous therapy was inhaled corticosteroids: 0.5 mg total daily dose given either once or twice daily in divided doses (maximum daily dose: 1 mg). If previous therapy was oral corticosteroids: 1 mg total daily dose given either as 0.5 mg twice a day or 1 mg daily (maximum daily dose: 1 mg).

DOSAGE: Pulmicort Turbuhaler

Prevention or treatment of asthma.

Children, over 6 years, if previous therapy was bronchodilators alone: 200 mcg twice a day, not to exceed 400 mcg twice a day. **Children, over 6 years, if previous therapy was inhaled corticosteroids:** 200 mcg twice a day, not to exceed 400 mcg twice a day. **Children, over 6 years, if previous therapy was oral corticosteroids:** Do not give more than 400 mcg twice a day.

DOSAGE: Aqua Nasal Spray RHINOCORT AQUA

Seasonal and perennial allergic rhinitis.

Children, 6 years and older, initial: 1 spray/nostril (64 mcg/day) once daily. **Maximum:** 2 sprays/nostril (128 mcg/day) once daily for children 6–11 years and 4 sprays/nostril (256 mcg) once daily for children 12 years and older. Maximum benefit seen in 2 weeks. After the maximum effect is obtained, reduce the maintenance dose to the smallest amount required to control symptoms.

NEED TO KNOW

1. Avoid exposure to chickenpox or measles.
2. Pulmicort Respules may be used in children as young as 12 months. In symptomatic children not responding to nonsteroidal therapy, a starting dose of 250 mcg using Respules may be tried.
3. Administer Pulmicort Respules using a jet nebulizer connected to an air compressor with an adequate air flow, equipped with a mouthpiece or suitable face mask. Ultrasonic nebulizers are not suitable. Do not administer with other nebulizable medications.
4. Rinse mouth (especially children) and equipment thoroughly after each use to prevent oral fungal infections.
5. Maximum benefit usually not seen for 3–7 days, although a decrease in symptoms can be seen within 24 hr. Report if no improvement within 3 weeks.

6. Shake canister well before administering. Store valve down and away from areas of high humidity.
7. Prime unit before use with Pulmicort Turbuhaler. Store respules upright protected from light; gently shake before use, discard open envelopes after 2 weeks.
8. Prior to using nasal spray gently shake container and prime the pump by actuating 8 times. If not used for 2 consecutive days, reprime with 1 spray or until a fine mist appears. If not used for more than 14 days, rinse the applicator and reprime with 2 sprays or until a fine mist appears.

Calfactant

(kal-**FAK**-tant)

Rx: Infasurf.

C

CLASSIFICATION(S): Lung surfactant

USES: Prevention and treatment of respiratory distress syndrome in premature infants.

ACTION/KINETICS: Adsorbs rapidly to the surface of the air: liquid interface and modifies surface tension similarly to natural lung surfactant.

SIDE EFFECTS: Cyanosis, airway obstruction, bradycardia, reflux of surfactant into the endotracheal tube, requirement for manual ventilation. *PULMONARY HEMORRHAGE, INTRAVENTRICULAR HEMORRHAGE, INTRACRANIAL HEMORRHAGE, NECROTIZING ENTEROCOLITIS, SEPSIS.*

DOSAGE: Suspension, Intratracheal

Prophylaxis of respiratory distress syndrome at birth.

Instill 3 mL/kg of birth weight as soon as possible after birth. Give as 2 doses of 1.5 mL/kg each. Care and stabilization of the premature infant born with hypoxemia or bradycardia should precede calfactant therapy.

Treatment of respiratory distress syndrome within 72 hr of birth.

Instill 3 mL/kg of birth weight, given as 2 doses of 1.5 mL/kg.

Repeat doses of 3 mL/kg of birth weight may be given, up to a total of 3 doses 12 hr apart.

NEED TO KNOW

1. Begin calfactant prophylaxis as soon as possible, within 30 minutes after birth.
2. Give only through an endotracheal tube.
3. Does not require reconstitution. Do not dilute, sonicate, or shake. Gently swirl/agitate vial for redispersion. Drug does not have to be warmed before administration.
4. Monitor carefully; adjust oxygen therapy and ventilatory support in response to changes in respiratory status. Reposition infant between each dose.

Carbamazepine ■ D

(kar-bah-**MAYZ**-eh-peen)

Rx: Carbatrol, Epitol, Equetro, Tegretol, Tegretol XR.

CLASSIFICATION(S): Anticonvulsant, miscellaneous

USES: (1) Partial seizures with complex symptoms (psychomotor, temporal lobe). (2) Generalized tonic-clonic seizures. (3) Mixed seizure patterns that include the above, or other partial or generalized seizures. Carbamazepine is often a drug of choice.

ACTION/KINETICS: The anticonvulsant action is not known but may involve depressing activity in the nucleus ventralis anterior of the thalamus, resulting in a reduction of polysynaptic responses and blocking posttetanic potentiation. Due to the potentially serious blood dyscrasias, undertake a benefit-to-risk evaluation before the drug is instituted. **Peak serum levels:** 4–5 hr. **$t^{1/2}$ (serum):** 12–17 hr with repeated doses. **Therapeutic serum levels:** 4–12 mcg/mL for children. Metabolized in the liver by the CYP3A4 isozyme to the 10,11-epoxide, which is also active. **$t^{1/2}$, initial:** 25–65 hr but is reduced to 12–17 hr because the drug induces its own metabolism. Metabolites are excreted through the feces (28%) and urine (72%). **Plasma protein binding:** 76%.

SIDE EFFECTS: Dizziness, drowsiness, unsteadiness, headache, N&V, ataxia, somnolence, rash, diarrhea, dyspepsia, infection, pain. *APLASTIC ANEMIA, AGRANULOCYTOSIS, BONE MARROW DEPRESSION, ARRHYTHMIAS (INCLUDING AV BLOCK), STEVENS-JOHNSON SYNDROME, HEPATIC FAILURE.*

DOSAGE: Capsules, Extended-Release; Oral Suspension; Tablets; Tablets, Chewable; Tablets, Extended-Release

Anticonvulsant

Children, over 12 years, initial: 200 mg 2 times per day if using tablets or extended-release products or 100 mg (5 mL) 4 times per day of the suspension. **Titration:** For tablets or suspension, increase at weekly intervals of no more than 200 mg/day using a 3- or 4-times per day regimen. For extended-release formulations, increase at weekly intervals of no more than 200 mg/day using a 2 times per day regimen. **Maintenance:** For all formulations, adjust to minimum effective dose, usually 800–1,200 mg/day. **Maximum daily dose, all formulations:** 12 to 15 years up to 1,000 mg/day. **Children, 6–12 years, initial:** 100 mg 2 times per day if using tablets or extended-release formulations or 50 mg (2.5 mL) 4 times per day of the suspension. **Titration:** For tablets or suspension, increase at weekly intervals of no more than 100 mg/day using a 3- or 4-times per day regimen. For extended-release formulations, increase at weekly intervals of no more than 100 mg/day using a 2 times per day regimen. **Maintenance:** For all formulations, adjust to minimum effective dose, usually 400–800 mg/day. **Maximum daily dose:** For tablets or suspension, 1,000 mg/day; for capsules, 35 mg/kg/day. **Children, younger than 6 years, initial:** 10–20 mg/kg/day in 2 to 3 divided doses if using tablets and 10–20 mg/kg/day in 4 divided doses if using the suspension. **Titration:** For tablets or suspension, increase weekly to achieve optimal clinical response given 3–4 times per day. **Maintenance:** For all formulations, usually optimal responses are achieved at daily doses less than 35 mg/kg. **Maximum daily dose:** For all formulations, 35 mg/kg/day.

NEED TO KNOW

1. To convert from tablets to suspension: give same number of mg/day in smaller, more frequent doses (e.g., tablets 2 times per day to suspension 3 times per day).
2. Convert from conventional tablets to extended-release tablets: give same total daily milligram dose of extended-release drug.
3. A given dose of suspension will produce higher peak levels than same dose given as the tablet; thus, start with low doses in children 6–12 years, increase slowly to avoid unwanted side effects.
4. If must discontinue due to side effects, abrupt withdrawal may lead to seizures or status epilepticus.
5. Take with meals to reduce GI upset.
6. Extended-release capsules may be opened and beads sprinkled over a teaspoon of applesauce or other similar food products. Do not crush/chew capsules or contents. May take with/without meals.

Cefaclor

(**SEF**-ah-klor)

Rx: Ceclor, Raniclor.

B

CLASSIFICATION(S): Cephalosporin, second generation

USES: **Capsules, Chewable Tablets, Oral Suspension:** (1) Otitis media due to *Streptococcus pneumoniae, Hemophilus influenzae, Streptococcus pyogenes*, and staphylococci. (2) Pharyngitis and tonsillitis caused by *S. pyogenes*. (3) Lower respiratory tract infections (including pneumonia) due to *S. pneumoniae, H. influenzae,* and *S. pyogenes*. (4) UTIs (including pyelonephritis and cystitis)

caused by *Escherichia coli, Proteus mirabilis, Klebsiella* species, and coagulase-negative staphylococci.
ACTION/KINETICS: **Peak serum levels:** 5–15 mcg/mL after 1 hr. **t½: PO,** 36–54 min. Well absorbed from GI tract.
SIDE EFFECTS: N&V, diarrhea, abdominal pain, GI upset, headache, yeast infection of the mouth or vagina.

DOSAGE: Capsules; Oral Suspension; Tablets, Chewable

All uses.

Children: 20 mg/kg/day in divided doses q 8 hr. May double dose in more serious infections, otitis media, or for infections caused by less susceptible organisms. For otitis media and pharyngitis, the total daily dose may be divided and given q 12 hr. Do not exceed a total dose of 2 grams/day.

NEED TO KNOW

1. Safety in infants less than 1 month of age not established.
2. Continue administration for a minimum of 48–72 hr after fever abates or after evidence of bacterial eradication has been obtained. For β-hemolytic streptococcal infections, continue treatment for at least 10 days as a prophylaxis for rheumatic fever or glomerulonephritis.
3. Refrigerate suspension after reconstitution; discard after 2 weeks.
4. Report any rash, adverse response, or lack of improvement after 48–72 hr.

Cefdinir
(**SEF**-dih-near)
Rx: Omnicef.

B

CLASSIFICATION(S): Cephalosporin, third generation
USES: **Children:** (1) Community-acquired pneumonia or acute exacerbations of chronic bronchitis. (2) Acute maxillary sinusitis. (3) Uncomplicated skin and skin structure infections.

(4) Pharyngitis/tonsillitis. **Children, 6 months through 12 years:** (1) Acute bacterial otitis media. (2) Pharyngitis/tonsillitis. (3) Uncomplicated skin and skin structure infections. *NOTE:* The suspension is approved for use for all infections in children indicated above.

ACTION/KINETICS: Interferes with the final step in cell wall formation (inhibition of mucopeptide biosynthesis), resulting in unstable cell membranes that undergo lysis. Also, cell division and growth are inhibited. **Maximum plasma levels:** 2–4 hr. **$t_{1/2}$, elimination:** 1.7 hr. Excreted through the urine.

SIDE EFFECTS: Diarrhea, N&V, vaginal moniliasis/vaginitis, headache, abdominal pain, rash.

DOSAGE: Capsules

Community-acquired pneumonia, uncomplicated skin and skin structure infections.

Children, age 13 and older: 300 mg q 12 hr for 10 days.

Acute exacerbations of chronic bronchitis, acute maxillary sinusitis, or pharyngitis/tonsillitis.

Children, age 13 and older: 300 mg q 12 hr for 5–10 days or 600 mg q 24 hr for 10 days for acute exacerbations of chronic bronchitis or pharyngitis/tonsillitis. Alternatively, 300 mg twice a day for 5 days for acute exacerbations of chronic bronchitis.

DOSAGE: Oral Suspension

Acute bacterial otitis media or pharyngitis/tonsillitis.

Children, 6 months through 12 years: 7 mg/kg q 12 hr for 5–10 days or 14 mg/kg q 24 hr for 10 days.

Uncomplicated skin and skin structure infections.

Children, 6 months through 12 years: 7 mg/kg q 12 hr for 10 days.

Acute maxillary sinusitis.

Children, 6 months through 12 years: 7 mg/kg q 12 hr or 14 mg/kg q 24 hr for 10 days.

NEED TO KNOW

1. Safety and efficacy have not been determined in infants less than 6 months of age.
2. For children, age 6 months through 12 years, the total daily dose for all infections is 14 mg/kg, up to a maximum of 600 mg/day. Except for skin infections, once-daily dosing for 10 days is as effective as twice-daily dosing.
3. The dosage of oral suspension for children is:
   - **9 kg (20 lb):** 2.5 mL q 12 hr or 5 mL q 24 hr of 125 mg/5 mL formulation.
   - **18 kg (40 lb):** 5 mL q 12 hr or 10 mL q 24 hr of 125 mg/5 mL formulation; or, 2.5 mL q 12 hr or 5 mL q 24 hr of 250 mg/5 mL formulation.
   - **27 kg (60 lb):** 7.5 mL q 12 hr or 15 mL q 24 hr of 125 mg/5 mL formulation; or, 3.75 mL q 12 hr or 7.5 mL q 24 hr of 250 mg/5 mL formulation.
   - **36 kg (80 lb):** 10 mL q 12 hr or 20 mL q 24 hr of 125 mg/5 mL formulation; or, 5 mL q 12 hr or 10 mL q 24 hr of 250 mg/5 mL formulation.
   - **Greater or equal to 43 kg (95 lb):** 12 mL q 12 hr or 24 mL q 24 hr of 125 mg/5 mL formulation; or, 6 mL q 12 hr or 12 mL q 24 hr of 250 mg/5 mL formulation.
4. Take without regard to food.
5. May give suspension in iron fortified infant formula without losing potency.
6. Report if diarrhea persistent, exceeds 4 episodes/day, accompanied by abdominal pain. Consume adequate fluids to prevent dehydation.
7. Stools may be discolored red; should subside.

Cefixime oral
(seh-**FIX**-eem)
Rx: Suprax.

B

CLASSIFICATION(S): Cephalosporin, third generation
USES: (1) Uncomplicated UTIs. (2) Otitis media. (3) Pharyngitis and tonsillitis. (4) Acute bronchitis and acute exacerbations of chronic bronchitis. (5) Uncomplicated cervical or urethral gonorrhea due to *N. gonorrhoeae*.
ACTION/KINETICS: Stable in the presence of beta-lactamase enzymes. **Peak serum levels:** 2–6 hr. **$t_{1/2}$:** Averages 3–4 hr. About 50% excreted unchanged in the urine and approximately 10% in the bile.
SIDE EFFECTS: N&V, diarrhea/loose stools, abdominal pain, dyspepsia, flatulence.

DOSAGE: Oral Suspension

All uses.

Children: Either 8 mg/kg once daily or 4 mg/kg q 12 hr. Give the adult dose to children greater than 50 kg or over 12 years (adult dose: 400 mg once daily or 200 mg q 12 hr).

NEED TO KNOW

1. Safe use in infants less than 6 months old not established.
2. Continue therapy for at least 10 days when treating *S. pyogenes*.
3. Use the following pediatric doses if using the 100 mg/5 mL suspension: **6.25 kg:** For a daily dose of 50 mg, give 2.5 mL; **12.5 kg:** For a daily dose of 100 mg, give 5 mL; **18.75 kg:** For a daily dose of 150 mg, give 7.5 mL; **25 kg:** For a daily dose of 200 mg, give 10 mL; **31.25 kg:** For a daily dose of 250 mg, give 12.5 mL; **37.5 kg:** For a daily dose of 300 mg, give 15 mL.
4. Use the following pediatric dose if using the 200 mg/5 mL suspension: **6.25 kg:** For a daily dose of 50 mg, give 1.25 mL; **12.5 kg:** For a daily dose of 100 mg, give 2.5 mL; **18.75 kg:**

For a daily dose of 150 mg, give 3.75 mL; **25 kg:** For a daily dose of 200 mg, give 5 mL; **31.25 kg:** For a daily dose of 250 mg, give 6.25 mL; **37.5 kg:** For a daily dose of 300 mg, give 7.5 mL.

5. Once reconstituted, keep suspension at room temperature or under refrigeration; discard after 14 days.
6. Once-a-day dosing should be taken at same time each day.

Cefprozil
(**SEF**-proh-zill)
Rx: Cefzil.

B

CLASSIFICATION(S): Cephalosporin, second generation
USES: (1) Pharyngitis and tonsillitis due to *Streptococcus pyogenes.* (2) Acute bacterial sinusitis due to *Streptococcus pneumoniae, Staphylococcus aureus, Haemophilus influenzae*, and *Moraxella catarrhalis.* (3) Otitis media caused by *S. pneumoniae, H. influenzae,* and *M. catarrhalis.* (4) Uncomplicated skin and skin structure infections due to *S. aureus* and *S. pyogenes.* (5) Secondary bacterial infection of acute bronchitis and acute bacterial exacerbation of chronic bronchitis due to *S. pneumoniae, H. influenzae,* and *M. catarrhalis.*
ACTION/KINETICS: **t½, after PO:** 78 min. 60% is recovered in the urine unchanged.
SIDE EFFECTS: N&V, diarrhea, abdominal pain, yeast infection of mouth or vagina.

DOSAGE: Oral Suspension; Tablets

Pharyngitis, tonsillitis.

Children, over 13 years: 500 mg q 24 hr for at least 10 days (for *S. pyogenes* infections, give 10 or more days). **2–12 years:** 7.5 mg/kg q 12 hr for at least 10 days (for *S. pyogenes* infections, give 10 or more days).

Acute sinusitis.

Children, over 13 years: 250 mg q 12 hr or 500 mg q 12 hr for 10 days. Use the higher dose for moderate to severe infections. **6 months–12 years:** 7.5 mg/kg q 12 hr or 15 mg/kg q 12 hr for 10 days. Use the higher dose for moderate to severe infections.

Secondary bacterial infections of acute bronchitis and acute bacterial exacerbation of chronic bronchitis.

Children, over 13 years: 500 mg q 12 hr for 10 days.

Uncomplicated skin and skin structure infections.

Children, over 13 years: Either 250 mg q 12 hr, 500 mg q 24 hr, or 500 mg q 12 hr (all for a duration of 10 days); **2–12 years:** 20 mg/kg q 24 hr for 10 days.

Otitis media.

Children, 6 months–12 years: 15 mg/kg q 12 hr for 10 days.

NEED TO KNOW

1. To enhance palatability/adherence, a suspension is available in a bubble-gum flavor.
2. Take as directed with/without food; food decreases stomach upset. Complete entire prescription, do not stop if feeling better. Refrigerate suspension and shake well before using; discard after 14 days.
3. Report lack of response, rash, diarrhea; may occur after therapy completed.

Cetirizine hydrochloride **B**

(seh-**TIH**-rah-zeen)

OTC: Zyrtec.

CLASSIFICATION(S): Antihistamine, second generation, piperazine

USES: (1) Relief of symptoms associated with seasonal allergic rhinitis due to ragweed, grass, and tree pollens in children over 6 years. (2) Perennial allergic rhinitis due to allergens such as dust

mites, animal dander, and molds in children over 6 years.
(3) Uncomplicated skin manifestations of chronic idiopathic urticaria in children over 6 years. Significantly reduces the occurrence, severity, and duration of hives and significantly reduces pruritus.
ACTION/KINETICS: Potent H_1-receptor antagonist. Protects against histamine-induced bronchospasm; low to negligible anticholinergic and sedative activity. Rapidly absorbed after PO administration. Food delays the time to peak serum levels. **t½:** 8.3 hr. Excreted mostly unchanged (95%) in the urine; 10% is excreted in the feces.
SIDE EFFECTS: Somnolence, dry mouth, fatigue, pharyngitis, dizziness, possible agressive reactions. *CONVULSIONS.*

DOSAGE: Syrup; Tablets; Tablets, Chewable

Seasonal or perennial allergic rhinitis, chronic urticaria.

Children, 12 years and older, initial: Depending on the severity of the symptoms, 5 or 10 mg (most common initial dose) once daily. **6–11 years:** 5 or 10 mg once daily, depending on severity of symptoms.

NEED TO KNOW

1. Use of antihistamines is not recommended in children less than 6 years.
2. May take with or without food; can vary time of administration based on need.
3. May cause dry mouth, fatigue; report adverse effects that prevent taking medications. Increase fluid intake to thin secretions.
4. Review allergens that trigger symptoms (ragweed, dust mites, molds, animal dander, etc.) and how to control/avoid contact.

Chlorpheniramine maleate **B**

(klor-fen-**EAR**-ah-meen)

OTC: Syrup: Aller-Chlor. **Tablets, Chewable:** Chlo-Amine. **Tablets:** Allergy Relief. **Tablets, Extended-Release:** Chlor-Trimeton Allergy 8 Hour and 12 Hour. **Rx: Caplets:** ED-CHLOR-TAN. **Capsules, Extended-Release Sustained-Release:** ODALL AR. **Oral Suspension:** Pediox-S.

CLASSIFICATION(S): Antihistamine, first generation, alkylamine

USES: Allergic rhinitis, including sneezing; itchy, watery eyes; itchy throat, and runny nose due to hay fever and other upper respiratory allergies.

ACTION/KINETICS: Moderate anticholinergic and low sedative activity. **Onset:** 15–30 min. **$t_{1/2}$:** 21–27 hr. **Time to peak effect:** 6 hr. **Duration:** 3–6 hr.

SIDE EFFECTS: Constipation, diarrhea, dizziness, drowsiness, dry mouth/nose/throat, headache, anorexia, N&V, anxiety, insomnia, GI upset, asthenia.

DOSAGE: Syrup; Tablets; Tablets, Chewable

Allergic rhinitis.

Children, over 12 years: 4 mg q 4–6 hr, not to exceed 24 mg in 24 hr; **6–12 years:** 2 mg (break 4-mg tablets in half) q 4–6 hr, not to exceed 12 mg in 24 hr.

DOSAGE: Caplets

Allergic rhinitis.

Children, 12 years and older: 8 mg q 12 hr, up to 16–24 mg/day; **6–12 years:** Consult a provider.

DOSAGE: Capsules, Extended-Release; Capsules, Sustained-Release

Allergic rhinitis.

Children, over 12 years: 8 or 12 mg q 12 hr, up to 16 or 24 mg/day; **6–12 years:** 8 mg at bedtime or during the day as indicated.

DOSAGE: Oral Suspension

Allergic rhinitis.

Children, 6–12 years: 2–4 mg (2.5–5 mL) q 12 hr; **over 12 years:** 4–8 mg (5–10 mL) q 12 hr.

DOSAGE: Tablets, Extended-Release

Allergic rhinitis.

Children, over 12 years: 8 mg q 8–12 hr or 12 mg q 12 hr, not to exceed 24 mg in 24 hr.

NEED TO KNOW

1. Do not use in children 6 years or younger.
2. Take as directed with a full glass of water. Food delays absorption.
3. Anticipate dry mouth and use appropriate remedies.

Clofarabine

(klo-**FAIR**-ah-been)

Rx: Clolar.

D

CLASSIFICATION(S): Antineoplastic, antimetabolite

USES: Acute lymphoblastic leukemia (ALL) in clients 1–21 years with relapsed or refractory ALL after at least 2 prior regimens.

ACTION/KINETICS: The drug inhibits DNA synthesis by decreasing cellular deoxynucleotide triphosphate pools through inhibition of ribonucleotide reductase, and by terminating DNA chain elongation and inhibiting repair through incorporation into the DNA chain by competitive inhibition of DNA polymerases. **$t^{1/2}$, terminal:** 5.2 hr. From 49–60% is excreted in the urine unchanged.

SIDE EFFECTS: Headache, dermatitis, pruritus, diarrhea, abdominal pain, N&V, anorexia, epistaxis, fatigue, pyrexia, rigors, flushing, hypotension, erythema, petechiae, constipation, febrile neutropenia, edema, pain in limb, cough, pain.

DOSAGE: IV Infusion

Acute lymphoblastic leukemia.

Children, 1–21 years: 52 mg/m^2 daily infused over 2 hr for 5 consecutive days. Repeat treatment cycle following recovery or return to baseline organ function (about every 2–6 weeks).

NEED TO KNOW

1. To prevent incompatibilities, do not administer any other medication through same IV line.
2. To reduce effects of tumor lysis/other side effects, give continuous IV fluids throughout the 5 days of clofarabine administration. The use of prophylactic steroids (e.g., hydrocortisone, 100 mg/m^2 on days 1 through 3) may prevent S&S of systemic inflammatory response syndrome or capillary leak.
3. Ensure adequate hydration, give continuous IV fluids during 5 days of clofarabine.
4. Report any dizziness, lightheadedness, fainting, reduced urine output. May experience vomiting/diarrhea; follow measures to prevent dehydration—take medications as directed.
5. If BP drops during therapy and rebounds, resume therapy but at a lower dose. If drop in BP requires medication therapy, stop therapy and continue supportive measures until stabilized.

Cromolyn sodium

B

(**CROH**-moh-lin)

OTC: Nasalcrom. **Rx:** Crolom, Cromolyn Sodium Ophthalmic Solution, Gastrocrom, Intal.

CLASSIFICATION(S): Antiasthmatic, antiallergic

USES: **Aerosol/Inhalation Solution:** (1) Prophylactic and adjunct in the management of bronchial asthma in clients who have a significant bronchodilator-reversible component to their airway obstruction. (2) Prophylaxis of acute bronchospasms induced by exercise, toluene diisocyanate, known allergens, or environmental pollutants. **Nasal, OTC:** Prophylaxis and treatment of allergic rhinitis, including children 2 years and older, due to airborne pollens from trees, grasses, or ragweed and by mold, animals, and dust. **PO:** Mastocytosis (improves symptoms including diarrhea, flushing, headaches, vomiting, urticaria, nausea, abdominal pain, and itching).

ACTION/KINETICS: Acts locally to inhibit the degranulation of sensitized mast cells that occurs after exposure to certain antigens. Prevents the release of histamine, slow-reacting substance of anaphylaxis, and other endogenous substances causing hypersensitivity reactions. After inhalation, some drug is absorbed systemically. **t½:** 81 min; from lungs: 60 min. About 50% excreted unchanged through the urine and 50% through the bile.

SIDE EFFECTS: **After PO/aerosol use:** Bronchospasm (maybe severe), cough, nasal congestion, pharyngeal irritation, wheezing. *BRONCHOSPASM, ANAPHYLAXIS.*

DOSAGE: Solution for Inhalation

Prophylaxis of bronchial asthma.

Children, over 2 years, initial: 20 mg inhaled 4 times per day at regular intervals.

Prophylaxis of exercise-induced bronchospasm.

Inhale 20 mg of the nebulizer solution no more than 1 hr (the shorter the interval between the dose and exercise, the better the effect) before anticipated exercise. Repeat as required for protection during prolonged exercise.

DOSAGE: Aerosol Spray

Management of bronchial asthma.

Children, 5 years and older, initial: 2 metered sprays inhaled 4 times per day at regular intervals. Do not exceed this dose.

Prophylaxis of acute bronchospasm.

Inhalation of 2 metered dose sprays 10–15 min (but not more than 60 min) before exposure to precipitating factor.

DOSAGE: Nasal Solution (OTC)

Allergic rhinitis.

Children, 2 years and older: 1 spray in each nostril 3–6 times per day at regular intervals q 4–6 hr. Maximum effect may not be seen for 1–2 weeks.

DOSAGE: Oral Concentrate

Mastocytosis.

Children, 13 years and older: 200 mg (i.e., 2 ampules) 4 times per day 30 min before meals and at bedtime; **2–12 years:** 100 mg (i.e., 1 ampule) 4 times per day 30 min before meals and at bedtime. If relief is not seen within 2–3 weeks, dose may be increased, but should not exceed 40 mg/kg/day. **Maintenance:** Reduce dose to minimum amount to maintain client with minimum symptoms.

NEED TO KNOW

1. Safety and efficacy have not been established for the aerosol in children under 5 years old, or for the nebulizer in children under 2 years old.
2. Reserve use in children under 2 years old to severe disease in which potential benefits clearly outweigh potential risks.
3. Continue corticosteroid dosage when initiating cromolyn therapy. If improvement occurs, taper the steroid dosage slowly.
4. Institute only after acute episode is over, when airway is clear and able to inhale adequately.
5. Do not discontinue inhalation or nasal medication abruptly. Rapid withdrawal of the drug may precipitate an asthmatic attack, and concomitant corticosteroid therapy may require adjustment.

Desloratadine
(**des**-lor-**AT**-ah-deen)
Rx: Clarinex, Clarinex Reditabs.

C

CLASSIFICATION(S): Antihistamine, second generation, piperidine
USES: (1) Relief of nasal and nonnasal symptoms of seasonal allergic rhinitis in children 6 years and older. (2) Relief of nasal and nonnasal symptoms of perennial allergic rhinitis in children 6 years and older. (3) Symptomatic relief of chronic idiopathic pruritus and reduction in the number and size of hives in children 6 years and older.
ACTION/KINETICS: Long-acting selective histamine H_1-receptor antagonist. Low to no anticholinergic or sedative activity. **Maximum plasma levels:** About 3 hr. Metabolized to 3-hydroxydesloratadine which is also active. **t½, elimination:** 27 hr.
SIDE EFFECTS: Dizziness, drowsiness/somnolence, headache, fatigue, pharyngitis, myalgia, dry mouth/nose/throat.

DOSAGE: Syrup; Tablets; Tablets, Rapidly Disintegrating
Chronic idiopathic urticaria, perennial/seasonal allergic rhinitis.
Children, over 12 years: 5 mg once daily (10 mL of the syrup); **6–11 years:** 2.5 mg once daily (5 mL of the syrup).

NEED TO KNOW
1. Antihistamines are not recommended for use in children less than 6 years.
2. May be taken without regard to meals.
3. Do not increase dose or dosing frequency as effectiveness is not increased and sleepiness may occur.

Dexmethylphenidate hydrochloride ■ C

(dex-**meth**-il-**FEN**-ah-dayt)

Rx: Focalin, Focalin XR, **C-II.**

CLASSIFICATION(S): CNS stimulant

USES: As part of a total program to treat attention deficit hyperactivity disorder in children 6 years and older.

ACTION/KINETICS: Drug is thought to block reuptake of norepinephrine and dopamine into the presynaptic neuron and increase the release of these neurotransmitters into the extraneuronal space. **Immediate-release tablets:** Rapidly absorbed; **maximum levels:** 1–1.5 hr. Food delays the time to maximum levels. **$t\frac{1}{2}$, elimination:** About 2.2 hr. **Extended-release capsules:** Produce a bimodal concentration-time profile about 4 hr apart. The drug is metabolized in the liver and excreted mainly in the urine.

SIDE EFFECTS: **Immediate-Release:** Abdominal pain, nausea, anorexia, fever, nervousness, anxiety, irritability, insomnia, weight loss, tachycardia, motor/vocal tics. **Extended-Release:** Headache, dyspepsia, decreased appetite, anxiety, dry mouth, pharyngolaryngeal pain, feeling jittery, dizziness.

DOSAGE: Tablets

Attention deficit hyperactivity disorder.

Children, new to methylphenidate: Initially, 2.5 mg twice a day of dexmethylphenidate. May adjust dose in 2.5–5 mg increments up to a maximum of 20 mg/day (10 mg twice a day). Dosage adjustments may be made at weekly intervals. **Those currently taking methylphenidate:** Start dexmethylphenidate at one-half the dose of racemic methylphenidate being used. Maximum recommended dose is 20 mg/day (10 mg twice a day). Clients currently using immediate-release dexmethylphenidate tablets may be switched to the same dose of extended-release dexmethylphenidate capsules.

DOSAGE: Capsules, Extended-Release

Attention deficit hyperactivity disorder.

Children, new to methylphenidate: 5 mg/day given once daily. Adjust dose, if needed, in 5 mg increments to a maximum of 20 mg/day. Observe the client for a sufficient period of time at a given dose to ensure that a maximum benefit has been reached before a dose increase is considered. Periodically assess need for the drug.

NEED TO KNOW

1. In psychotic children, worsening of symptoms of behavior disturbance and thought disorder may occur.
2. Give twice a day at least 4 hr apart, with/without food.
3. Discontinue drug if improvement is not seen after appropriate dosage adjustment over a 1-month period.
4. Take before/with breakfast and lunch to avoid interference with sleep. Take extended-release capsules once daily in the morning.
5. Take extended-release capsules whole or by sprinkling the contents on a small amount of applesauce. Do not crush, chew, or divide capsules. Consume the mixture with applesauce immediately; do not store for future use.
6. Therapy may be interrupted periodically ('drug holiday') to determine if it is still necessary in those responsive to therapy and in some to permit normal growth.

Dextroamphetamine sulfate ■ C

(dex-troh-am-**FET**-ah-meen)

Rx: Dexedrine, Dexedrine Spansules, Dextrostat, **C-II.**

CLASSIFICATION(S): CNS stimulant

USES: (1) As part of a total treatment program for attention deficit disorders with hyperactivity in children 3 to 16 years.
(2) Narcolepsy.

ACTION/KINETICS: Stronger CNS effects and weaker peripheral action than amphetamine. After PO, completely absorbed in 3 hr. **Duration: PO,** 4–24 hr; **$t_{1/2}$, children:** 6–8 hr. Excreted in urine. Acidification will increase excretion, while alkalinization will decrease it.

SIDE EFFECTS: Nausea, GI upset, cramps, anorexia, diarrhea, constipation, dry mouth, headache, nervousness, dizziness, insomnia, irritability, restlessness.

DOSAGE: Capsules, Sustained-Release; Tablets

Attention deficit disorders.

Children, 3–5 years: 2.5 mg/day initially; increase in increments of 2.5 mg/day at weekly intervals until optimum response reached. **6 years and older:** 5 mg once or twice daily initially; increase in increments of 5 mg/day at weekly intervals until optimum response reached. Dosage will rarely exceed 40 mg/day.

Narcolepsy.

Children, over 12 years: Initial: 10 mg/day; increase dose in increments of 10 mg/day at weekly intervals. Reduce dose if side effects occur. **6–12 years: Initial:** 5 mg/day; increase in increments of 5 mg at weekly intervals until optimum effect is reached, up to a maximum of 60 mg/day.

NEED TO KNOW

1. Not recommended for use in children less than 3 years.
2. Higher rates of serious CV events and sudden death are seen with amphetamine compared with methylphenidate in children.
3. Dosage for narcolepsy has not been determined in children less than 6 years.
4. Use of extended-release capsules for attention deficit disorders in children less than 6 years is not recommended.
5. Avoid late evening doses, especially with sustained-release capsules due to the possibility of insomnia.
6. When tablets are used for attention deficit disorder or narco-

lepsy, give first dose upon awakening with one or two additional doses given at intervals of 4–6 hr. Give the last dose 6 hr before bedtime.

7. Where possible interrupt drug administration occasionally to determine the need for continued therapy.

Dextromethorphan hydrobromide **C**
(dex-troh-meth-**OR**-fan)

OTC: Freezer Pops: PediaCare Children's Long-Acting Cough. **Gelcaps:** DexAlone, Robitussin CoughGels. **Liquid/Oral Solution:** Children's Pedia Care Long-Acting Cough, Creo-Terpin, Robitussin Maximum Strength Cough, Simply Cough, Vicks 44 Cough Relief. **Lozenges:** Hold DM, Scot-Tussin DM Cough Chasers, Trocal. **Oral Suspension, Extended-Release:** Delsym. **Strips, Orally Disintegrating:** TheraFlu Thin Strips Long-Acting Cough, Triaminic Thin Strips Long Acting Cough. **Syrup:** Creomulsion for Children, ElixSure Children's Cough, Robitussin Pediatric Cough, Silphen DM. **Rx: Suspension:** AeroTuss 12.

CLASSIFICATION(S): Antitussive, nonnarcotic

USES: Symptomatic relief of nonproductive cough due to colds or inhaled irritants.

ACTION/KINETICS: Selectively depresses the cough center in the medulla. Does not produce physical dependence or respiratory depression. Well absorbed from GI tract. **Onset:** 15–30 min. **Duration:** 3–6 hr.

SIDE EFFECTS: Dizziness, drowsiness, GI disturbances.

DOSAGE: Freezer Pops

Antitussive.

Children, 6 to less than 12 years: 2 freezer pops (50 mL), if needed, q 6–8 hr, up to 8 freezer pops (200 mL)/day.

DOSAGE: Gelcaps

Antitussive.

Children, 12 years and older: 30 mg q 6–8 hr, not to exceed 120 mg/24 hr. Do not use in children less than 12 years.

DOSAGE: Lozenges

Antitussive.

Children, 12 years and older: 5–15 mg q 1–4 hr, up to 120 mg/day; **6–12 years:** 5–10 mg q 1–4 hr, not to exceed 60 mg/day. Do not give to children under 6 years unless directed by provider.

DOSAGE: Liquid; Oral Solution; Syrup

Antitussive.

Children, 12 years and older: 10–20 mg q 4 hr or 30 mg q 6–8 hr, not to exceed 120 mg/day; **6–12 years:** 10 mg q 4 hr or 15 mg q 6–8 hr, up to 60 mg/day.

DOSAGE: Oral Suspension, Extended-Release

Antitussive.

Children, 12 years and older: 60 mg q 12 hr, up to 120 mg/day; **6–12 years:** 30 mg q 12 hr, up to 60 mg/day.

NEED TO KNOW

1. Do not use in children less than 6 years.
2. Use with caution in clients with nausea, vomiting, high fever, rash, or persistent headache.
3. Increasing the dose of dextromethorphan will not increase its effectiveness but will increase the duration of action.
4. Increase fluids to decrease thickness of secretions.

Diazepam

(dye-**AYZ**-eh-pam)

Rx: Diastat AcuDial, Diazepam Intensol, Valium, **C-IV.**

D

CLASSIFICATION(S): Antianxiety drug, benzodiazepine

USES: PO: (1) Management of anxiety disorders or for short-term relief of symptoms of anxiety. (2) Adjunct therapy in convulsive disorders; effectiveness as sole therapy has not been proven. (3) Adjunct for relief of skeletal muscle spasm caused by reflex spasm to local pathology (e.g., inflammation of muscles or joints or secondary to trauma). Also, spasticity due to upper motor neuron disorders (e.g., cerebral palsy, paraplegia). Athetosis. **Parenteral:** (1) Adjunct therapy in status epilepticus and severe recurrent convulsive seizures. (2) Treatment of tetanus. (3) Adjunct for the relief of skeletal muscle spasm due to reflex spasm caused by local pathology (e.g., inflammation of muscles or joints, secondary to trauma). Also, spasticity due to upper motor neuron disorders (e.g., cerebral palsy, paraplegia); athetosis. **Rectal gel:** Management of selective refractory clients with epilepsy who are stable on regimens of anticonvulsant drugs who require intermittent diazepam to control increased seizure activity.

ACTION/KINETICS: Reduces anxiety by increasing or facilitating the inhibitory neurotransmitter activity of GABA. The skeletal muscle relaxant effect may be due to enhancement of GABA-mediated presynaptic inhibition at the spinal level as well as in the brain stem reticular formation. **Onset: PO,** 30–60 min; **IM,** 15–30 min; **IV,** more rapid. **Peak plasma levels: PO,** 0.5–2 hr; **IM,** 0.5–1.5; **IV,** 0.25 hr. **Duration:** 3 hr. **t½:** 20–50 hr. Metabolized in the liver. Diazepam and metabolites are excreted through the urine. **Plasma protein binding:** 97–99%.

SIDE EFFECTS: Drowsiness (transient), ataxia, confusion.

DOSAGE: Oral Solution; Solution, Intensol; Tablets

Management and relief of anxiety disorders.

Children, initial: 1–2.5 mg 3–4 times per day; **then,** increase gradually as needed and tolerated. Not to be used in children less than 6 months of age.

Adjunct in skeletal muscle spasms.

Children: 0.12–0.8 mg/kg/24 hr divided 3 to 4 times per day.

Adjunct in convulsive disorders.

Children, at least 6 months of age, initial: 1–2.5 mg 3 or 4 times per day; **then,** increase dose gradually as needed and tolerated.

DOSAGE: IM; IV

Sedation or muscle relaxation.

Children: 0.04–0.2 mg/kg/dose q 2–4 hr up to a maximum of 0.6 mg/kg within an 8-hr period.

Tetanus.

Children, 5 years and older: 5–10 mg given q 3–4 hr, if needed. **Infants older than 30 days of age:** 1–2 mg IM or slowly IV given q 3–4 hr as needed.

Status epilepticus or severe recurrent convulsive seizures.

Children, at least 5 years: 1 mg q 2–5 min IV (preferred) up to a maximum of 10 mg. Repeat in 2–4 hr if needed. **Infants older than 30 days of age and younger than 5 years:** 0.2–0.5 mg by slow IV q 2–5 min up to a maximum of 5 mg. May be repeated in 2–4 hr if needed.

DOSAGE: Rectal Gel

Convulsive disorders.

Children, 12 years and older: 0.2 mg/kg; **6–11 years:** 0.3 mg/kg; **2–5 years:** 0.5 mg/kg. If needed, a second dose may be given 4–12 hr after the first dose. Do not treat more than 5 episodes/month or more than 1 episode q 5 days.

NEED TO KNOW

1. Do not give parenterally in children under 12 years.
2. Mix Intensol solution with beverages such as water, soda, and juices or soft foods such as applesauce or puddings. Use only

the calibrated dropper provided to withdraw drug; once withdrawn and mixed, use immediately.

3. Except for the deltoid muscle, absorption from IM sites is slow, erratic, and painful and not generally recommended.
4. EEG monitoring of seizures may be helpful.

Dicyclomine hydrochloride
(dye-**SYE**-kloh-meen)
Rx: Antispas, Bentyl, Byclomine, Di-Spaz, Dibent, Dilomine, Or-Tyl.

C

CLASSIFICATION(S): Cholinergic blocking drug
USES: Hypermotility and spasms of GI tract associated with irritable colon and spastic colitis, mucous colitis.
ACTION/KINETICS: Prevents acetylcholine from combining with postganglionic parasympathetic nerve receptors (muscarinic) resulting in decreased vagal impulses to the GI tract. Results in a decrease in GI motility. **t½, initial:** 1.8 hr; **secondary:** 9–10 hr.
SIDE EFFECTS: Dry mouth, N&V, constipation, urinary hesitancy/retention, headache, blurred vision. **Use of the syrup in infants less than 3 months of age:** *SEIZURES*, syncope, respiratory symptoms, fluctuations in pulse rate, *ASPHYXIA*, muscular hypotonia, *COMA*.

DOSAGE: Capsules; Syrup; Tablets
Hypermotility and spasms of GI tract.
Children, 6 months–2 years, syrup: 5–10 mg 3–4 times per day; **2 years and older:** 10 mg 3–4 times per day. The dose should be adjusted to need and incidence of side effects.

NEED TO KNOW
1. Take 30 min before meals and at bedtime, report lack of response, rash, skin eruption, or adverse effects.
2. Consume adequate fluids to prevent dehydration/constipation; may use sugarless candy/gum for dry mouth. Avoid

strenuous activity during hot conditions; heatstroke may occur.

Didanosine (ddI, dideoxyinosine) ■ B

(die-**DAN**-oh-seen)

Rx: Videx.

CLASSIFICATION(S): Antiviral, nucleoside reverse transcriptase inhibitor

USES: Videx: Use in combination with other antiretroviral drugs to treat HIV-1 infections. May be used in children over 2 weeks of age.

ACTION/KINETICS: After entering the cell, it is converted to the active dideoxyadenosine triphosphate (ddATP) by cellular enzymes. Due to the chemical structure of ddATP, its incorporation into viral DNA leads to chain termination and therefore inhibition of viral replication. Is broken down quickly at acidic pH; therefore, PO products contain buffering agents to increase the pH of the stomach. Food decreases the rate of absorption. Oral availability in children (about 25%). **$t\frac{1}{2}$, elimination:** 0.8 hr for children. Metabolized in the liver and excreted mainly through the urine.

SIDE EFFECTS: Diarrhea, N&V, headache, peripheral neurologic symptoms/neuropathy, abdominal pain, rash, pruritus, pancreatitis. *SEIZURES, HEMORRHAGE.*

DOSAGE: Capsule, Enteric-Coated; Powder for Oral Solution, Buffered; Powder for Pediatric Oral Solution; Tablets, Buffered (Chewable/Dispersible)

Children: 120 mg/m^2 2 times per day. Once-daily dosing may lower the virologic response; twice-daily dosing is preferred.

NEED TO KNOW

1. Opportunistic infections and other complications of HIV infec-

tion may continue to develop; thus, keep clients under close observation.

2. Administer all formulations 30 min before or 1 hr after meals.
3. To prepare powder for pediatric oral solution, mix the dry powder with purified water to an initial concentration of 20 mg/mL. The resulting solution is then mixed with antacid (e.g., Mylanta Double Strength Liquid, Extra Strength Maalox Plus Suspension, or Maalox TC Suspension) to a final concentration of 10 mg/mL. Shake this admixture thoroughly prior to use. May be stored in a tightly closed container, in the refrigerator for up to 30 days.
4. Report any symptoms of neuropathy (numbness, burning, or tingling in the hands or feet); drug should be discontinued until symptoms subside.
5. Report any abdominal pain and N&V immediately; may be clinical signs of pancreatitis. Stop drug and report; resume only after pancreatitis has been ruled out.
6. Chewable/dispersible buffered tablets contain 73 mg phenylalanine per 2-tablet dose.

Digoxin

(dih-**JOX**-in)

A

Rx: Digitek, Digoxin Injection Pediatric, Lanoxicaps, Lanoxin.

CLASSIFICATION(S): Cardiac glycoside

USES: (1) CHF, including that due to venous congestion, edema, dyspnea, orthopnea, and cardiac arrhythmia. May be drug of choice for CHF because of rapid onset, relatively short duration, and ability to be administered PO or IV. (2) Control of rapid ventricular contraction rate in clients with atrial fibrillation or flutter. (3) SVT. (4) Prophylaxis and treatment of recurrent paroxysmal atrial tachycardia with paroxysmal AV junctional rhythm.

ACTION/KINETICS: Increases the force and velocity of myocardial contraction (positive inotropic effect) by increasing the refractory

period of the AV node and increasing total peripheral resistance. Digoxin also decreases HR, decreases the rate of conduction, and increases the refractory period of the AV node due to an increase in parasympathetic tone and a decrease in sympathetic tone. **Onset:** PO, 0.5–2 hr; **time to peak effect:** 2–6 hr. **Duration:** Over 24 hr. **Onset, IV:** 5–30 min; **time to peak effect:** 1–4 hr. **Duration:** 6 days. **$t\frac{1}{2}$:** 30–40 hr. **Therapeutic serum level:** 0.5–2.0 ng/mL. **Plasma protein binding:** 20–25%.
SIDE EFFECTS: Tachycardia, headache, dizziness, mental disturbances, N&V, diarrhea, anorexia, blurred or yellow vision. Digoxin is extremely toxic and has caused *DEATH* even in clients who have received the drug for long periods of time. *DEATH MOST OFTEN RESULTS FROM VENTRICULAR FIBRILLATION.*

DOSAGE: Capsules

Digitalization: Slow.

Children: Digitalizing dosage is divided into three or more doses with the initial dose being about one-half the total dose; doses are given q 4–8 hr. **Children, 10 years and older:** 0.008–0.012 mg/kg. **5–10 years:** 0.015–0.03 mg/kg. **2–5 years:** 0.025–0.035 mg/kg. **1 month–2 years:** 0.03–0.05 mg/kg. **Neonates, full-term:** 0.02–0.03 mg/kg. **Neonates, premature:** 0.015–0.025 mg/kg.

Maintenance.

Premature neonates: 20–30% of total digitalizing dose divided and given in two to three daily doses. **Neonates to 10 years:** 25–35% of the total digitalizing dose divided and given in two to three daily doses.

DOSAGE: Elixir; Tablets

Digitalization: Slow.

Children: Digitalizing dose is divided into two or more doses and given at 6–8-hr intervals. **Children, 10 years and older, rapid or slow:** Same as adult dose (0.125–0.5 mg/day for 7 days). **5–10 years:** 0.02–0.035 mg/kg. **2–5 years:** 0.03–0.05

mg/kg. **1 month–2 years:** 0.035–0.06 mg/kg. **Premature and newborn infants to 1 month:** 0.02–0.035 mg/kg.

Maintenance.

Children: One-fifth to one-third the total digitalizing dose daily. *NOTE:* An alternate regimen (referred to as the "small-dose" method) is 0.017 mg/kg/day. This dose causes less toxicity.

DOSAGE: IV

Digitalization.

Children: Same as tablets.

NEED TO KNOW

1. Use with caution in newborn, term, or premature infants who have immature renal and hepatic function.
2. Be especially alert to cardiac arrhythmias in children.
3. Measure liquids precisely using calibrated dropper/syringe.
4. For clients being digitalized and for clients on maintenance dose digoxin:
   - With digitalization, monitor closely.
   - Observe and monitor for bradycardia/arrhythmias, count apical rate for at least 1 min before administering drug.
   - If client's HR is 90–110 bpm or if arrhythmia present; withhold drug and report.
5. Anticipate more than once-daily dosing in most children (up to age 10) related to higher metabolic activity.
6. When given to newborns, use cardiac monitor to identify early evidence of toxicity: excessive slowing of sinus rate, sinoatrial arrest, prolonged PR interval.
7. Take after meals to lessen gastric irritation.
8. Do not change brands; different preparations have variations in bioavailability and may cause toxicity or loss of effect.

Dimenhydrinate

(dye-men-**HY**-drih-nayt)

OTC: Liquid: Children's Dramamine, Dramamine. **Tablets:** Calm-X, Dramamine, Triptone. **Tablets, Chewable:** Dramamine, **Rx: Injection:** Dinate, Dramanate, Dymenate. **Liquid:** Dramamine.

CLASSIFICATION(S): Cholinergic blocking drug, antiemetic
USES: (1) Motion sickness, especially to relieve nausea, vomiting, or dizziness. (2) Vertigo.
ACTION/KINETICS: Antiemetic mechanism not known, but it does depress labyrinthine and vestibular function. Possesses anticholinergic activity. **Duration:** 3–6 hr.
SIDE EFFECTS: Drowsiness, confusion (especially in children), headache, dizziness, blurred/double vision.

DOSAGE: Liquid; Tablets; Tablets, Chewable

Motion sickness.

Children, 6–12 years: 25–50 mg q 6–8 hr, not to exceed 150 mg/day; **2–6 years:** 12.5–25 mg q 6–8 hr, not to exceed 75 mg/day.

DOSAGE: IM; IV

Children, over 2 years: 1.25 mg/kg (37.5 mg/m^2) 4 times per day, not to exceed 300 mg/day.

DOSAGE: IV

Children: 1.25 mg/kg (37.5 mg/m^2) in 10 mL of 0.9% sodium chloride given slowly over 2 min; may be repeated q 6 hr, not to exceed 300 mg/day.

NEED TO KNOW

1. Use of the injectable form is not recommended in neonates.
2. Adjust pediatric dosage per BSA.

3. Take at least 30 min before departure; may repeat before meals and upon retiring for motion sickness prevention.
4. May alter skin testing results; wait 72 hr after use.

Diphenhydramine hydrochloride

(dye-fen-**HY**-drah-meen)

B

OTC: Anti-Allergy/Anti-Cough. Capsules or Capsules, Soft Gel: Banophen, Benadryl Allergy Kapseals, Diphenhist, Genahist. **Liquid:** Scot-Tussin Allergy Relief Formula Clear. **Oral Solution:** Children's Pedia Care Nighttime Cough. **Strips, Oral Disintegrating:** Triaminic Thin Strips Cough & Runny Nose, Triaminic Thin Strips Multi-Symptoms. **Syrup:** Hydramine Cough, Silphen Cough. **Rx: Syrup:** Tusstat.

CLASSIFICATION(S): Antihistamine, second generation, ethanolamine

USES: (1) Hypersensitivity reactions (type I), including perennial and seasonal allergic rhinitis, vasomotor rhinitis, and sneezing caused by the common cold, allergic conjunctivitis caused by inhalant allergens and foods, mild uncomplicated allergic skin manifestations of urticaria and angioedema, amelioration of allergic reactions to blood or plasma, dermatographism, adjunctive anaphylactic therapy, uncomplicated allergic conditions of the immediated type. (2) Antitussive (syrup only).

ACTION/KINETICS: High sedative, anticholinergic, and antiemetic effects.

SIDE EFFECTS: Drowsiness, constipation, diarrhea, dizziness, dry mouth/nose/throat, headache, anorexia, N&V, anxiety, GI upset, asthenia.

DOSAGE: Capsules; Capsules, Soft Gel; Elixir; Liquid; Oral Solution; Syrup; Tablets; Tablets, Chewable; Tablets, Oral Disintegrating

Hypersensitivity reactions, motion sickness.

Children, 6–12 years: 12.5–25 mg PO 3–4 times per day, not to exceed 150 mg/day.

DOSAGE: Liquid

Antitussive.

Children, 12 years and older: 25–50 mg q 4 hr, not to exceed 300 mg in 24 hr; **6–12 years:** 12.5–25 mg q 4 hr, not to exceed 150 mg in 24 hr; **6 years and younger:** Do not use.

DOSAGE: Oral Solution

Antitussive.

Children, 6 to less than 12 years: 12.5 mg (5 mL) q 4 hr, up to 75 mg (30 mL)/day; **less than 6 years:** Do not use.

DOSAGE: Syrup

Antitussive.

Children, 6–12 years: 12.5 mg q 4 hr, not to exceed 75 mg/day; **2–6 years:** Do not use.

DOSAGE: IM (Deep); IV

Hypersensitivity reactions, motion sickness.

Children, 6 years and older: 1.25 mg/kg (or 37.5 mg/m^2) 4 times per day, not to exceed a total of 300 mg/day divided into 4 doses given IV at a rate not exceeding 25 mg/min or deep IM.

NEED TO KNOW

1. Do not use in children 6 years and younger.
2. With motion sickness, give full prophylactic dose 30 min prior to travel and 1–2 hr before exposures that precipitate sickness.
3. Do not exceed an IV rate of 25 mg/min.

4. May cause drowsiness; use caution until drug effects realized.
5. Stop therapy 72 to 96 hr before skin testing performed.

Dornase alfa recombinant

(**DOR**-nace **AL**-fah)

Rx: Pulmozyme.

B

CLASSIFICATION(S): Treatment of cystic fibrosis

USES: In clients with cystic fibrosis (CF) in conjunction with standard therapy to decrease the frequency of respiratory infections that require parenteral antibiotics and to improve pulmonary function.

ACTION/KINETICS: Dornase alfa hydrolyzes the DNA in sputum of clients with CF, thereby reducing sputum viscoelasticity and reducing infections.

SIDE EFFECTS: Pharyngitis, chest pain, rash, voice alteration, conjunctivitis, laryngitis. *APNEA*.

DOSAGE: Solution for Inhalation

Cystic fibrosis.

One 2.5-mg (2.5 mL) single-dose ampule inhaled once daily using a recommended nebulizer.

NEED TO KNOW

1. Safety and effectiveness of daily use have not been demonstrated in clients with forced vital capacity (FVC) of less than 40% of predicted, or for longer than 12 months.
2. Approved nebulizers include the disposable jet nebulizer Hudson T U-draft II, disposable jet nebulizer Marquest Acorn II in conjunction with a Pulmo-Aide compressor, and the reusable PARI LC Jet+ nebulizer in conjunction with the PARI PRONEB compressor.
3. Do not dilute or mix with other drugs in nebulizer.
4. Product does not contain a preservative; thus, once opened, entire ampule must be used or discarded.

5. Must be administered on a daily schedule to obtain full benefits. Must continue standard therapies for CF (e.g., chest PT, antibiotics, bronchodilators, oral and inhaled corticosteroids, enzyme supplements, vitamins, and analgesics) during therapy.

Doxycycline calcium

D

(dox-ih-**SYE**-kleen)

Rx: Vibramycin.

Doxycycline hyclate

Rx: Atridox, Doryx, Doxy 100 and 200, Periostat, Vibra-Tabs, Vibramycin.

Doxycycline monohydrate

Rx: Adoxa, Monodox, Vibramycin.

CLASSIFICATION(S): Antibiotic, tetracycline

USES: (1) Gram-negative organisms. *Haemophilus ducreyi, Francisella tularensis, Yersenia pestis, Bartonella bacilliformis, Campylobacter fetus, Vibrio cholerae, Brucella* species (with streptomycin) to treat brucellosis, *Calymmatobacterium granulomatis*. (2) *Rickettsiae*. (3) *Mycoplasma pneumoniae* (e.g., respiratory tract infections). (4) *Chlamydia trachomatis*. (5) *Chlamydia psittaci*. (6) *Borellia recurrentis*. (7) *Ureaplasma urealyticum*. (8) For the following infections following susceptibility testing as resistance has been documented: *Escherichia coli, Enterobacter aerogenes, Acinetobacter* species, *Haemophilus influenzae, Klebsiella* species, *Streptococcus pneumoniae, Shigella* species. (9) Adjunct to amebicides for acute intestinal amebiasis. (10) Reduce incidence or progression of anthrax (including inhalational anthrax) following exposure to aerosolized *Bacillus anthracis*. (11) Prophylaxis of malaria due to *Plasmodium falciparum* in short-term travelers (less than 4 months) to areas with chloroquine and/or pyrimethamine-sulfadoxine resistant strains.

ACTION/KINETICS: Inhibits protein synthesis by binding to the ribosomal 30S subunit. Blocks binding of aminoacyl transfer RNA to the messenger RNA complex. Cell wall synthesis is not inhibited. **t½:** 15–25 hr; 30–42% excreted unchanged in urine. High lipid solubility. **Plasma protein binding:** From 80–95%.

SIDE EFFECTS: Anorexia, N&V, diarrhea, dizziness, headache, rashes.

DOSAGE: Capsules; Capsule, Enteric-Coated; IV; Oral Suspension; Syrup; Tablets; Tablets, Delayed-Release

Infections.

Children, over 8 years (45 kg or less): First day, 4.4 mg/kg in 2 doses; **then,** 2.2–4.4 mg/kg/day in divided doses depending on severity of infection. Children over 45 kg should receive the adult dose **(first day:** 100 mg q 12 hr; **maintenance:** 100 mg/day).

Prophylaxis of malaria.

Children, over 8 years: 2 mg/kg/day up to 100 mg/day. Begin 1–2 days before travel to endemic area and continue during travel and for 4 weeks after returning.

Anthrax, inhalation, post-exposure.

Children, weighing 45 kg or more: 100 mg q 12 hr for 60 days; **less than 45 kg:** 2.2 mg/kg q 12 hr for 60 days.

DOSAGE: IV Infusion Only

Infections.

Children, over 8 years, up to 45 kg: 4.4 mg/kg on day 1 in 1 or 2 infusions; **then,** 2.2–4.4 mg/kg given as 1 or 2 infusions, depending on severity of the infection. **Over 45 kg:** Use adult dose (200 mg IV on day 1 given in 1 or 2 infusions; **then,** 100–200 mg, depending on severity of condition).

NEED TO KNOW

1. Do not use in children less than 8 years old. In children up to 8 years tetracycline may cause permanent discoloration of the teeth.

2. When used for streptococcal infections, continue therapy for 10 days.
3. Malaria prophylaxis can begin 1–2 days before travel begins, during travel, and for 4 weeks after leaving the malarial area.
4. Avoid rapid IV administration.
5. May take with food; take caps with a full glass of water to prevent esophageal ulceration and remain upright for 45 min.
6. Avoid direct exposure to sunlight and wear protective clothing and sunscreens when exposed.
7. Take entire prescription; do not stop if symptoms subside. Report adverse effects or lack of response.

Ethosuximide

(eth-oh-**SUCKS**-ih-myd)

Rx: Zarontin.

C

CLASSIFICATION(S): Anticonvulsant, succinimide

USES: Absence (petit mal) seizures. May be given concomitantly with other anticonvulsants if other types of epilepsy are manifested with absence seizures.

ACTION/KINETICS: Acts by depressing the motor cortex and by raising the threshold of the CNS to convulsive stimuli. Rapidly absorbed from the GI tract. **Peak serum levels:** 3–7 hr. **$t^{1/2}$, children:** 30 hr. Steady serum levels reached in 7–10 days. **Therapeutic serum levels:** 40–100 mcg/mL. Both inactive metabolites and unchanged drug are excreted in the urine.

SIDE EFFECTS: Drowsiness, dizziness, blurred vision, GI upset, anorexia, headache, hiccoughs. *AGRANULOCYTOSIS, STEVENS-JOHNSON SYNDROME.*

DOSAGE: Capsules; Syrup

Absence seizures.

Children, over 6 years, initial: 250 mg twice a day; the dose may be increased by 250 mg/day at 4–7-day intervals until seizures are controlled or until total daily dose reaches 1.5 grams. **Under 6 years, initial:** 250 mg/day; dosage may be increased by 250 mg/day every 4–7 days until control is established or total daily dose reaches 1 gram.

NEED TO KNOW

1. Take with meals to minimize GI upset. Do not stop abruptly; may increase severity and frequency of seizures.
2. Any persistent fever, swollen glands, and bleeding gums may signal a blood dyscrasia and require reporting. Report significant weight loss, rash, joint pain, fever.
3. Alert family to the possibility of transient personality changes, hypochondriacal behavior, and aggressiveness, which should be reported.

Etodolac
(ee-toh-**DOH**-lack)

C

CLASSIFICATION(S): Nonsteroidal anti-inflammatory

USES: Relief of signs and symptoms of juvenile rheumatoid arthritis.

ACTION/KINETICS: Anti-inflammatory effect likely due to inhibition of cyclo-oxygenase which results in decreased prostaglandin synthesis. **Time to peak levels:** 1–2 hr. **Onset of analgesic action:** 30 min; **duration:** 4–12 hr. **t½:** 7.3 hr. The drug is metabolized by the liver and metabolites are excreted through the kidneys (72%) and feces (16%). **Plasma protein binding:** More than 99%.

SIDE EFFECTS: Dizziness, asthenia/malaise, abdominal pain/cramps, diarrhea, nausea, flatulence.

DOSAGE: Tablets, Extended-Release

Juvenile rheumatoid arthritis (use Extended-Release Tablets).

Children, 6–16 years (based on body weight). 20–30 kg: 1–400 mg tablet once daily. **31–45 kg:** 1–600 mg tablet once daily. **46–60 kg:** 2–400 mg tablets once daily. **Greater than 60 kg:** 2–500 mg tablets once daily.

NEED TO KNOW

1. Do not use in clients in whom etodolac, aspirin, or other NSAIDs have caused asthma, rhinitis, urticaria, or other allergic reactions.
2. Seek the lowest dose and longest dosing interval for each client.
3. Take with milk or food to decrease GI upset.
4. May cause dizziness or drowsiness; avoid activities requiring alertness until drug effects realized.
5. Report any unusual bruising/bleeding, rash, yellow skin discoloration, dark/tarry stools, or lack of response.

6. Stop drug and report, sudden weight gain, loss of BP control, swelling in extremities, blood in stools or urine.
7. Use protection if exposed and avoid prolonged sun exposure.

Famotidine

(fah-**MOH**-tih-deen)

B

OTC: Pepcid AC, Pepcid AC Maximum Strength.

Rx: Pepcid, Pepcid RPD.

CLASSIFICATION(S): Histamine H_2 receptor blocking drug

USES: PO/Injection, Rx: (1) Pathologic hypersecretory conditions such as Zollinger-Ellison syndrome or multiple endocrine adenomas. (2) Treatment, up to 6 weeks, of GERD, including ulcerative disease diagnosed by endoscopy or erosive esophagitis. (3) Treatment, up to 8 weeks, of active, benign gastric ulcer. **PO, OTC:** (1) Relief of heartburn associated with indigestion and sour stomach. (2) Prevent heartburn associated with acid indigestion and sour stomach due to certain foods and beverages. **IV:** (1) Some hospitalized clients with pathological hypersecretory conditions or intractable ulcers. (2) Alternative to PO dosage forms for short-term use in those who are unable to take PO medication.

ACTION/KINETICS: Competitive inhibitor of histamine H_2 receptors leading to inhibition of gastric acid secretion. Both basal and nocturnal gastric acid secretion stimulated by food or pentagastrin are inhibited. **Peak plasma levels:** 1–3 hr. **t½:** 2.5–3.5 hr. **Onset:** 1 hr. **Duration:** 10–12 hr. From 25 to 30% of a PO dose is eliminated through the kidney unchanged; from 65 to 70% of an IV dose is excreted through the kidney unchanged.

SIDE EFFECTS: Headache, dizziness, diarrhea, constipation, N&V, anxiety, confusion.

DOSAGE: Rx: Oral Suspension; Tablets; Tablets, Oral Disintegrating

Peptic ulcers.

Children, 1–16 years: 0.5 mg/kg/day at bedtime or divided twice a day up to 40 mg/day. Individualize dose based on clinical response and/or gastric/esophogeal pH and endoscopy.

GERD with or without esophagitis, including erosions and ulcerations.

Children, 1–16 years: 1 mg/kg/day PO divided twice daily, up to 40 mg twice daily.

GERD.

Children, less than 1 year, initial: 0.5 mg/kg/dose of the oral suspension for up to 8 weeks. Give once daily (i.e., 0.5 mg/kg) in children younger than 3 months of age and twice daily (i.e., 0.5 mg/kg twice daily) to children from 3 months to younger than 1 year.

DOSAGE: IV; IV Infusion

Hospitalized clients with hypersecretory conditions, duodenal ulcers, gastric ulcers; unable to take PO medication.

Children, 1–16 years: Individualize. **Initial:** 0.25 mg/kg given over 2 or more minutes or as a 15-min infusion q 12 hr up to 40 mg/day. **Initial, infants less than 1 year:** 0.5 mg/kg/dose once daily, for up to 8 weeks in infants younger than 3 months of age and 0.5 mg/kg/dose twice daily, for up to 8 weeks in infants 3 months to younger than 1 year of age. These clients should also receive conservative measures (e.g., thickened feedings).

DOSAGE: OTC: Gelcaps ; Tablets ; Tablets, Chewable

Relief and prevention of heartburn, acid indigestion, and sour stomach.

Children, over 12 years, for prevention: 10 or 20 mg 15–60 min before eating food or drinking a beverage expected to cause symptoms. **Relief (acute therapy):** 10 mg or 20 mg with water. **Maximum dose:** 20 mg/24 hr. Not to be used continuously for more than 2 weeks unless medically prescribed.

NEED TO KNOW

1. Use of IV famotidine in children younger than 1 year has not been adequately studied. Do not give the OTC product to children younger than 12 years unless otherwise directed.
2. The oral suspension may be substituted for tablets for any use.
3. Take with food at night.
4. May take with antacids for pain relief. Drug may cause dizziness, headaches, and anxiety; use caution with activities requiring mental alertness and report if symptoms persist.

Fexofenadine hydrochloride

(fex-oh-**FEN**-ah-deen)

Rx: Allegra, Allegra ODT.

C

CLASSIFICATION(S): Antihistamine, second generation, piperidine

USES: (1) Seasonal allergic rhinitis, including sneezing; rhinorrhea; itchy nose, throat, or palate; and itchy, watery, and red eyes in children 6 years and older. (2) Uncomplicated skin manifestations of chronic idiopathic urticaria in children 6 years and older.

ACTION/KINETICS: An H_1-histamine receptor blocker. Low to no sedative or anticholinergic effects. **Onset:** Rapid. **Peak plasma levels:** 2.6 hr. **t½, terminal:** 14.4 hr. Approximately 90% of the drug is excreted through the feces (80%) and urine (10%) unchanged.

SIDE EFFECTS: Headache, dyspepsia, coughing, URTI, viral infection, back pain.

DOSAGE: Oral Suspension; Tablets; Tablets, Oral Disintegrating

Seasonal allergic rhinitis; chronic idiopathic urticaria.

Children, over 12 years: 60 mg twice a day or 180 mg once daily; **6–11 years:** 30 mg twice a day. *NOTE:* **Children, over 12 years with decreased renal function, initial:** 60 mg once daily; **6–11 years with decreased renal function, initial:** 30 mg once daily.

NEED TO KNOW

1. Use is not recommended in children less than 6 years.
2. Take as directed; do not crush, break or chew sustained release tabs.
3. May take with food to decrease stomach upset.
4. May experience headaches, sore throat, nausea, and dysmenorrhea.
5. Avoid prolonged or excessive exposure to direct or artificial sunlight.
6. Report if symptoms intensify or do not improve after 48 hr.

Fluconazole
(flew-**KON**-ah-zohl)
Rx: Diflucan.

C

CLASSIFICATION(S): Antifungal
USES: (1) Oropharyngeal and esophageal candidiasis. (2) Serious systemic candidal infection (including UTIs, peritonitis, candidemia, disseminated candidiasis, and pneumonia). (3) Cryptococcal meningitis and candidal infections.
ACTION/KINETICS: A highly selective inhibitor of fungal cytochrome P450 and sterol C-14 alpha-demethylation. There is a decrease in cell wall integrity and extrusion of intracellular material, leading to death. **Peak plasma levels:** 1–2 hr. **Steady-state levels:** 5–10 days after 50–400 mg given once a day. **t½:** 30 hr, which allows for once daily dosing. Penetrates all body fluids at steady state. Eighty percent of the drug is excreted unchanged by the kidneys.
SIDE EFFECTS: **Following single doses:** Headache, nausea, abdominal pain, diarrhea. ANGIOEDEMA, ANAPHYLAXIS (RARE). **Following multiple doses:** Nausea, headache, skin rash, vomiting, abdomi-

nal pain. *SERIOUS HEPATIC REACTIONS, SEIZURES, STEVENS-JOHNSON SYNDROME, TOXIC EPIDERMAL NECROLYSIS.*

DOSAGE: IV; Oral Suspension; Tablets

Oropharyngeal or esophageal candidiasis.

Children, first day: 6 mg/kg; **then,** 3 mg/kg once daily for a minimum of 14 days (for oropharyngeal candidiasis) or 21 days (for esophageal candidiasis).

Systemic candidiasis (e.g., candidemia, disseminated candidiasis, and pneumonia).

Children: 6–12 mg/kg/day.

Acute cryptococcal meningitis.

Children, first day: 12 mg/kg; **then,** 6 mg/kg once daily for 10 to 12 weeks after CSF culture is negative.

Maintenance to prevent relapse of cryptococcal meningitis in clients with AIDS.

Children: 6 mg/kg once daily.

NEED TO KNOW

1. Efficacy has not been determined in children less than 6 months of age.
2. Daily dose is same for PO and IV administration.
3. Do not exceed continuous IV infusion rate of 200 mg/hr. Check site frequently for extravasation/necrosis.
4. Do not add supplementary medication to IV bag.
5. Report rash, N&V, diarrhea, yellowing of skin, clay-colored stools, dark urine, lack of response, or persistent side effects; may need to be discontinued.
6. Avoid prolonged or excessive exposure to direct or artificial sunlight.

Flunisolide
(flew-**NISS**-oh-lyd) ■ C

Rx: Inhalation Aerosol: AeroBid, AeroBid-M. **Intranasal:** Nasarel.

Flunisolide Hemihydrate

Rx: AeroSpan.

CLASSIFICATION(S): Glucocorticoid

USES: **AeroBid, AeroBid-M, AeroSpan:** (1) Maintenance treatment of asthma as prophylactic therapy in children, 6 years and older. (2) For those who require systemic corticosteroids where adding flunisolide may reduce or eliminate the need for PO corticosteroids. **Nasarel:** Relief and management of nasal symptoms of seasonal and perennial allergic rhinitis.

ACTION/KINETICS: Minimal systemic effects with intranasal use. Significant first-pass after inhalation; rapidly metabolized by the liver. Several days may be required for full beneficial effects. **t½:** 1–2 hr. Metabolized in the liver and excreted by the feces (50%) and urine (50%).

SIDE EFFECTS: **After use of the aerosol:** N&V, diarrhea, flu, sore throat, headache, cold symptoms, nasal congestion, URTI, unpleasant taste. **After use of the solution/spray:** Burning, dryness, nasal irritation, sneezing, throat irritation/itching.

DOSAGE: Aerosol (AeroBid, AeroBid-M) FLUNISOLIDE

Chronic asthma.

Children, 5–15 years: 2 inhalations twice daily for a total daily dose of 1 mg.

DOSAGE: Solution/Spray NASAREL

Allergic rhinitis.

Children, 6–14 years: 1 spray in each nostril 3 times per day or 2 sprays in each nostril twice a day. **Maximum dose:** 4 sprays in each nostril daily. **Maintenance, children:** Smallest dose necessary to control symptoms.

DOSAGE: Aerosol (AeroSpan) FLUNISOLIDE HEMIHYDRATE

Chronic asthma.

Children, 12 years and older, initial: 160 mcg twice daily, not to exceed 320 mcg twice daily; **6–11 years, initial:** 80 mcg twice daily, not to exceed 160 mcg twice daily.

NEED TO KNOW

1. Safety and efficacy in children less than 6 years have not been determined.
2. When initiating in those receiving systemic corticosteroids, use aerosol concomitantly with the systemic steroid for 1 week. Then, slowly withdraw the systemic corticosteroid over several weeks.
3. If nasal congestion is present, use a decongestant before administration to ensure drug reaches site of action.
4. If beneficial effects do not occur within 3 weeks, discontinue therapy.
5. Before use, prime the nasal spray by pushing down on the pump 5 or 6 times until a fine mist appears. If the pump has not been used for 5 days or more, the spray must be primed again.
6. Mild nasal bleeding may occur; this is usually transient.

Fluticasone furoate

(flu-**TIH**-kah-sohn) ■ C

Rx: Veramyst.

Fluticasone propionate

Rx: Cream, Lotion, Ointment: Cutivate. **Aerosol**: Flovent. **Powder for Inhalation**: Flovent Rotadisk. **Spray**: Flonase.

CLASSIFICATION(S): Glucocorticoid

USES: Fluticasone furoate; Intranasal: Symptoms of seasonal and perennial allergic rhinitis in children 2 years and older. **Fluticasone propionate; Respiratory Inhalation:** Maintenance treatment of asthma as prophylactic therapy in children 4 years and older (Flovent HFA, Flovent Rotadisk, and Flovent Diskus). **Intranasal:** As needed to manage nasal symptoms of seasonal and perennial allergic and nonallergic rhinitis in children over 4 years (Flonase). Atopic dermatitis in children as young as 3 months.

ACTION/KINETICS: Anti-inflammatory due to ability to inhibit prostaglandin synthesis. Also inhibits accumulation of macrophages and leukocytes at sites of inflammation as well as inhibits phagocytosis and lysosomal enzyme release. **Onset:** Approximately 12 hr. **Maximum effect:** May take several days. **$t_{1/2}$:** About 3.1 hr. Absorbed drug is metabolized in the liver by CYP3A4 and excreted in the feces (>95%) and urine (<5%). **Plasma protein binding:** About 91%.

SIDE EFFECTS: Flonase: Headache, pharyngitis, epistaxis, nasal burning/irritation, N&V, asthma symptoms, cough.
Flovent: Throat irritation, URTI, sinusitis/sinus infection, oral candidiasis, headache, fever. *ANAPHYLAXIS, POSSIBLE SEVERE FATAL ASTHMA.*

DOSAGE: Aerosol FLUTICASONE PROPIONATE

Asthma.

Children, over 4 years, initial: 88 mcg twice a day (maximum: 440 mcg twice a day) if previous therapy was bronchodilators alone; 88–220 mcg twice a day (maximum: 440 mcg twice a day) if previous therapy was inhaled corticosteroids; and, 440 mcg twice a day (maximum: 880 mcg twice a day) if previous therapy was oral corticosteroids.

DOSAGE: Powder for Inhalation FLOVENT ROTADISK

Prevention of asthma.

Children, 12 years and older: 100 mcg twice a day (maximum: 500 mcg twice a day) if previous therapy was bronchodilators alone; 100–250 mcg twice a day (maximum: 500 mcg twice a day) if previous therapy was inhaled corticosteroids; and, 500 (using the Diskus) to 1,000 mcg twice a day (maximum: 1,000 mcg twice a day) if previous therapy was oral corticosteroids. **4–11 years:** 50 mcg twice a day (maximum: 100

mcg twice a day) if previous therapy was bronchodilators alone or inhaled corticosteroids.

DOSAGE: Nasal Spray FLONASE

Allergic rhinitis.

Children, 4 years and older, initial: 100 mcg (1 spray/nostril once a day). If no response to 100 mcg, may use 200 mcg/day (2 sprays/nostril). Once control achieved, decrease dose to 100 mcg (1 spray/nostril) daily. Do not exceed a dose of 200 mcg/day. The spray is not recommended for children under 4 years.

DOSAGE: Spray, Intranasal Suspension FLUTICASONE FUROATE

Seasonal and perennial allergic rhinitis.

Children, 12 years and older, initial: 110 mcg once daily given as 2 sprays (27.5 mcg/spray) in each nostril. Titrate to the minimum effective dose to reduce the possibility of side effects. When the maximum benefit has been reached, reduce the dose to 55 mcg (1 spray in each nostril) once daily. **2–11 years, initial:** 55 mcg once daily given as 1 spray (27.5 mcg/spray) in each nostril. Children not responding adequately to the 55 mcg dose may use 110 mcg (2 sprays/nostril) once daily. Once symptoms have been controlled, decrease the dose to 55 mcg daily.

NEED TO KNOW

1. Clients on immunosuppressant drugs, such as corticosteroids, are more susceptible to infections.
2. For Flonase, initially prime the pump with 6 actuations before use or after a period of non-use of 1 week or more.
3. Before use of Flonase, shake gently. Discard the Flonase bottle when the labeled number of actuations has been used.
4. Do not exceed prescribed dose, it may take several days to achieve full benefits. Take at regular intervals to ensure effectiveness.
5. Do not interrupt therapy if side effects evident; notify provider as drug may require slow withdrawal. The dosage should also be slowly reduced if S&S of hypercorticism or adrenal suppres-

sion occur such as depression, lassitude, joint and muscle pain; report if evident, especially when replacing systemic corticosteroids with topical.

Formoterol fumarate ■ C

(for-**MOH**-tur-all)

Rx: Foradil Aerolizer, Perforomist.

CLASSIFICATION(S): Sympathomimetic, direct-acting

USES: Inhalation Powder in Capsules: (1) Long-term maintenance treatment of asthma and to prevent bronchospasms in children 5 years and older who have reversible obstructive airway disease, including nocturnal asthma, who require regular treatment with inhaled, short-acting, beta$_2$-agonists. (2) Acute prevention of exercise-induced bronchospasm in children 5 years and older. Used on an occasional, as needed, basis.

ACTION/KINETICS: Long-acting selective beta$_2$-agonist. Acts locally in the lung as a bronchodilator. Acts in part by increasing cyclic AMP levels causing relaxation of bronchial smooth muscle and inhibition of release of mediators of immediate hypersensitivity, especially from mast cells. When inhaled, is rapidly absorbed into the plasma, reaching maximum plasma levels within 5 min. Metabolized in the liver to inactive metabolites. Excreted in the urine and feces. **t$^{1/2}$, terminal:** 10 hr.

SIDE EFFECTS: Viral infection, bronchitis, chest infection/pain, dyspnea, tremor, dizziness, dry mouth, insomnia. *ANAPHYLAXIS.*

DOSAGE: Capsules for use in Aerolizer FORADIL AEROLIZER

Maintenance treatment of asthma and to prevent bronchospasm.

Children, over 5 years: Inhale contents of one 12 mcg-capsule q 12 hr (morning and evening) using the Aerolizer inhaler. Do not exceed 24 mcg/day. If symptoms appear between doses, use an inhaled short-acting beta$_2$-agonist for immediate relief.

Prevention of exercise-induced bronchospasm.

Children, 12 years and older: Inhale contents of one 12-mcg capsule at least 15 min before exercise. Give on an occasional, as needed, basis. When used for prevention, protection may last up to 12 hr; do not use additional doses for 12 hr.

NEED TO KNOW

1. Long-acting $beta_2$-adrenergic agonists may increase the risk of asthma-related death.
2. Use only with Aerolizer inhaler, do not take orally.
3. Can be used together with short-acting $beta_2$-agonists, inhaled or systemic corticosteroids, and theophylline.
4. If taking formoterol in twice-daily doses for asthma, do not take additional doses for exercise-induced bronchospasms.
5. A satisfactory response to formoterol does not eliminate the need for continued treatment with an anti-inflammatory drug.
6. Formoterol is not a substitute for inhaled or oral corticosteroids.
7. Do not expose capsules to moisture; handle with dry hands. Do not wet or wash the Aerolizer inhaler; keep dry. Always use the new Aerolizer inhaler with each refill.
8. Report any unusual side effects, loss of control of breathing patterns, or intolerance to therapy.

Gabapentin
(**gab**-ah-**PEN**-tin)
Rx: Gabarone, Neurontin.

C

CLASSIFICATION(S): Anticonvulsant, miscellaneous

USES: (1) Treatment of partial seizures with and without secondary generalization in clients 12 years and older. (2) Adjunct to treat partial seizures in children 3–12 years.

ACTION/KINETICS: Is related chemically to GABA but does not interact with GABA receptors. **t½:** 5–7 hr. Excreted unchanged through the urine. Adjust dosage in those with impaired renal function.

SIDE EFFECTS: Dizziness, somnolence, peripheral edema, ataxia, nystagmus, tremor. *CONVULSIONS, INTRACRANIAL HEMORRHAGE, SUICIDAL TENDENCIES, SUDDEN UNEXPLAINED DEATHS.*

DOSAGE: Capsules; Oral Solution; Tablets

Partial seizures with and without secondary generalization.

Children, 12 years and older: Dose range of 900–1,800 mg/day in three divided doses using 300 or 400 mg capsules or 600 or 800 mg tablets. **Initial dose:** 300 mg 3 times per day; dose may be increased, as needed, up to 1,800 mg/day. Doses up to 2,400 and 3,600 mg/day have been well tolerated for short periods.

Adjunctive therapy for partial seizures in children.

Children, 3–12 years, initial: 10–15 mg/kg/day in 3 divided doses. Attain effective dose by titration over 3 days. Effective dose in clients 5 years and older is 25–35 mg/kg/day and in children 3 and 4 years is 40 mg/kg/day; give in divided doses 3 times per day.

NEED TO KNOW

1. Use in children 3–12 years is associated with various neuropsychiatric side effects (e.g., emotional lability, hostility including aggression, thought disorder including concentration problems and change in school performance, hyperkinesia).
2. Safety and efficacy have not been determined in children less than 3 years.
3. Do not allow 12 hr to pass between any 2 doses using the 3 times per day daily regimen.
4. The first dose on day 1 may be taken at bedtime to minimize somnolence, dizziness, fatigue, and ataxia.
5. When drug therapy is discontinued or supplemental therapy added, do so gradually over at least 1 week.

6. May be taken with or without food. Do not chew or crush; use half tablets within several days of breaking the scored tablet.
7. If trouble swallowing, may open capsule and mix with applesauce or juice. Mix only one dose at a time just before taking it.
8. May cause dizziness, fatigue, drowsiness, incoordination, and eye twitching.
9. Report any seizures, visual changes, unusual bruising/bleeding, loss of effect, new/unusual side effects. Do not stop suddenly with prolonged therapy.

Guaifenesin

(gwye-**FEN**-eh-sin) **C**

OTC: Oral Liquid: Mucinex Children's, Robitussin, Scot-Tussin Expectorant, Siltussin SA. **Syrup:** Altarussin, Guiatuss. **Tablets, Extended-Release:** Humabid Maximum Strength, Mucinex. **Granules:** Mucinex Mini-Melts Children's, Mucinex Mini-Melts Junior Strength.
Rx: Oral Liquid: Organidin NR. **Tablets:** Liquidbid, Organidin NR.

CLASSIFICATION(S): Expectorant
USES: (1) Dry, nonproductive cough due to colds and minor upper respiratory tract infections when there is mucus in the respiratory tract. (2) To loosen phlegm and thin bronchial secretions.
ACTION/KINETICS: May increase the output of fluid from the respiratory tract by reducing the viscosity and surface tension of respiratory secretions, thereby removing accumulated secretions from the upper and lower airway. Readily absorbed from the GI tract. Rapidly metabolized and excreted in the urine. **t½:** 1 hr.
SIDE EFFECTS: N&V, GI discomfort.

DOSAGE: Granules

Expectorant.

Children, 12 years and older: 200–400 mg (2 to 4 of the 100 mg/packet strength) q 4 hr, up to 6 doses/day; **6 to less than 12 years:** 100–200 mg (1 to 2 of the 100 mg/packet strength or 2 to 4 of the 50 mg/packet strength) q 4 hr, up to 6 doses/day.

DOSAGE: Oral Liquid; Syrup; Tablets

Expectorant.

Children, 12 years and older: 200–400 mg q 4 hr, not to exceed 2,400 mg/day; **6–11 years:** 100–200 mg q 4 hr, not to exceed 1,200 mg/day; **less than 6 years: Do not use.**

DOSAGE: Tablets, Extended-Release

Expectorant.

Children, 12 years and over: 600–1,200 mg q 12 hr, not to exceed 2,400 mg/day.

NOTE: The liquid dosage forms may be more suitable for children 6–12 years.

NEED TO KNOW

1. Do not use in chronic cough (e.g., due to asthma or emphysema), cough accompanied by excess secretions.
2. Do not use in children under age 6.
3. Mucinex is not recommended for children less than 12 years.
4. Take tablets with a full glass of water.
5. Notify provider if symptoms persist more than 1 week, recur, or accompanied by a persistent headache, fever, or rash.

Hydrochlorothiazide **B**

(**hy**-droh-klor-oh-**THIGH**-ah-zyd)

Rx: Ezide, Hydro-Par, HydroDIURIL, Microzide Capsules.

CLASSIFICATION(S): Diuretic, thiazide

USES: Hypertension.

ACTION/KINETICS: Promote the excretion of sodium and chloride, and thus water, by the distal renal tubule. Also increases ex-

cretion of potassium and to a lesser extent bicarbonate. The antihypertensive activity is thought to be due to direct dilation of the arterioles, as well as to a reduction in the total fluid volume of the body and altered sodium balance. **Onset:** 2 hr. **Peak effect:** 4–6 hr. **Duration:** 6–12 hr. **t½:** 5.6–14.8 hr. Hydrochlorothiazide is not metabolized but is eliminated rapidly by the kidney.
SIDE EFFECTS: Orthostatic hypotension, hypokalemia, weakness, headache, diarrhea, dizziness, gastric upset/irritation/cramping. *TOXIC EPIDERMAL NECROLYSIS, STEVENS-JOHNSON SYNDROME, ANAPHYLACTIC REACTIONS, RESPIRATORY DISTRESS INCLUDING PNEUMONITIS AND PULMONARY EDEMA.*

DOSAGE: Capsules; Oral Solution; Tablets

Antihypertensive.

Children, under 6 months: 3.3 mg/kg/day in two doses; **up to 2 years:** 12.5–37.5 mg/day in two doses; **2–12 years:** 37.5–100 mg/day in two doses.

NEED TO KNOW

1. Give twice a day at 6–12-hr intervals.
2. To prevent nighttime urinary frequency take in the a.m. with a glass of orange juice. May take with food if GI upset. Report side effects or lack of response.
3. May cause dizziness; change positions slowly and avoid activities that require mental alertness until drug effects realized.

Hydroxyzine hydrochloride

(hy-**DROX**-ih-zeen)

Hydroxyzine pamoate

Rx: Vistaril.

C

CLASSIFICATION(S): Antianxiety drug, nonbenzodiazepine
USES: (1) Sedation when used as premedication and following general anesthesia. (2) Anxiety and tension associated with psychoneurosis and as an adjunct in organic diseases in which anxiety is manifested. (3) Pruritus due to allergic conditions such as

chronic urticaria or atopic or contact dermatoses; also, histamine-mediated pruritus.

ACTION/KINETICS: Action may be due to a suppression of activity in selected key regions of the subcortical areas of the CNS. Significant sedative and antiemetic effects and moderate anticholinergic activity. Rapidly absorbed. **Onset:** 15–30 min. **$t^{1/2}$:** 3 hr. **Duration:** 4–6 hr. Metabolized by the liver and excreted through the urine.

SIDE EFFECTS: Sedation, drowsiness, tiredness, dizziness, disturbed coordination, drying/thickening of oral and other respiratory secretions, stomach upset.

DOSAGE: Capsules; Oral Suspension; Syrup; Tablets

Sedation.

Children: 0.6 mg/kg.

Anxiety and tension.

Children, over 6 years: 50–100 mg/day in divided doses; **less than 6 years:** 50 mg/day in divided doses.

Pruritus.

Children, over 6 years: 50–100 mg/day in divided doses; **less than 6 years:** 50 mg/day in divided doses.

DOSAGE: IM HYDROXYZINE HYDROCHLORIDE

Sedation.

Children: 0.6 mg/kg.

NEED TO KNOW

1. Inject IM only. In children, inject into the midlateral muscles of the thigh. In infants and small children, to minimize sciatic nerve damage, use the periphery of the upper outer quadrant of the gluteal region only when necessary (e.g., burn clients). Do not make IM injections into the lower and mid-third of the upper arm.
2. Careful mouth care with frequent rinsing, sucking hard candy, chewing sugarless gum, and increased fluid intake may relieve S&S of dry mouth.

3. Wait and evaluate sedative effects of drug before performing tasks that require mental alertness.

Hyoscyamine sulfate

(high-oh-**SIGH**-ah-meen) **C**

Rx: Anaspaz, Cystospaz, ED-SPAZ, IB-Stat, Levbid, Levsin, Levsin Drops, Levsin/SL, Levsinex Timecaps, Mar-Spas, Neosol, NuLev, Symax Duotab, Symax FasTab, Symax-SL, Symax-SR.

CLASSIFICATION(S): Cholinergic blocking drug
USES: (1) To control gastric secretion, visceral spasm, and hypermotility in spastic colitis, spastic bladder, cystitis, pylorospasm, and associated abdominal cramps. (2) Relieve symptoms in functional intestinal disorders (e.g., mild dysenteries and diverticulitis), infant colic, biliary colic. (3) Irritable bowel syndrome (e.g., irritable colon, spastic colon, mucous colitis, acute enterocolitis, functional GI disorders). (4) Treat poisoning by anticholinesterase agents. (5) Preoperative medication to reduce salivary, tracheobronchial, and pharyngeal secretions.
ACTION/KINETICS: Acts by blocking the action of acetylcholine at the postganglionic nerve endings of the parasympathetic nervous system. **t½:** 3.5 hr for tablets, 7 hr for extended-release capsules, and 9 hr for extended-release tablets. Majority of the drug is excreted in the urine unchanged.
SIDE EFFECTS: Dry mouth, drowsiness, flushing of face, headache, blurred vision, photosensitivity, constipation, decreased sweating, thirst.

DOSAGE: Capsules, Extended-Release; Tablets, Extended-Release; Tablets, Timed-Release

Children, over 12 years: 0.375–0.750 mg q 12 hr, not to exceed 1.5 mg in 24 hr.

DOSAGE: Tablets; Tablets, Sublingual

Children, over 12 years: 0.125–0.25 mg q 4 hr or as needed, not to exceed 1.5 mg in 24 hr.

DOSAGE: Tablets, Oral Disintegrating

0.125 mg: Children, over 12 years: 1 or 2 tablets q 4 hr, up to 12/day or 2 tablets 4 times per day. **2 to less than 12 years:** ½–1 tablet q 4 hr, up to 6 per day.

0.25 mg: Children, over 12 years: ½–1 tablet 3–4 times per day, 30 min to 1 hr before meals and at bedtime. This dosage form is not recommended for children under 12 years old.

DOSAGE: Elixir

Children, over 12 years: 0.125 mg–0.25 mg (5–10 mL) q 4 hr, not to exceed 1.5 mg (60 mL) in 24 hr. **2 to 12 years: 10 kg:** 1.25 mL (0.031 mg) q 4 hr; **20 kg:** 2.5 mL (0.062 mg) q 4 hr; **40 kg:** 3.75 mL (0.093 mg) q 4 hr; **50 kg:** 5 mL (0.125 mg) q 4 hr.

DOSAGE: Drops

Children, over 12 years: 0.125–0.25 mg (5–10 mL) q 4 hr, not to exceed 1.5 mg (12 mL) in 24 hr. **2 to 12 years:** 0.031–0.125 mg (0.22–1 mL) q 4 hr or as needed, not to exceed 0.75 mg (6 mL) in 24 hr. **Under 2 years: 3.4 kg:** 4 drops q 4 hr, not to exceed 24 drops in 24 hr; **5 kg:** 5 drops q 4 hr, not to exceed 30 drops in 24 hr; **7 kg:** 6 drops q 4 hr, not to exceed 36 drops in 24 hr; **10 kg:** 8 drops q 4 hr, not to exceed 48 drops in 24 hr.

DOSAGE: Oral Spray

Children, 12 years and younger: 1–2 mL (1 or 2 sprays) q 4 hr as needed, up to 12 mL/day (12 sprays/day).

DOSAGE: Injection

Preanesthetic medication.

Children, over 2 years: 0.005 mg/kg 30–60 min prior to the time of induction of anesthesia. May also be given at the time the preanesthetic sedative or narcotic is given.

During surgery to reduce drug-induced bradycardia.

Children, over 2 years: Increments of 0.125 mg (0.25 mL) IV repeated as needed.

Reverse neuromuscular blockade.

Children, over 2 years: 0.2 mg (0.4 mL) for every 1 mg neostigmine or equivalent dose of physostigmine or pyridostigmine.

NEED TO KNOW

1. Take as prescribed; avoid antacids within 1 hr of taking drug (decreases effectiveness).
2. Avoid excessive temperatures and activity; drug impairs heat regulation and may decrease perspiration, which may cause fever, heat prostration, or stroke.
3. Stop drug and report any mental confusion, impaired gait, disorientation, or hallucinations.

Ibuprofen ■ **B,D**
(eye-byou-**PROH**-fen)

OTC: Oral Drops: Infants' Motrin, PediaCare Fever. **Suspension**: Children's Advil, Children's Motrin, PediaCare Fever, Pediatric Advil Drops. **Tablets, Chewable**: Children's Advil, Children's Motrin, Junior Strength Advil, Junior Strength Motrin.

Ibuprofen lysine

Rx: NeoProfen.

CLASSIFICATION(S): Nonsteroidal anti-inflammatory

USES: Chewable Tablets, Junior Strength Tablets, Oral Suspension, Oral Drops, Children: (1) Temporary reduction of fever. (2) Relief of minor aches and pains due to colds, flu, sore throat, headaches, and toothaches. **Ibuprofen lysine. Rx (IV):** To close clinically significant patent ductus arteriosus in infants whose gestational age is 32 weeks or less, weight is 500–1,500 grams, and the condition cannot be managed through usual therapy (e.g., diuretics, fluid restriction, respiratory support).

ACTION/KINETICS: Anti-inflammatory effect is likely due to inhibition of cyclo-oxygenase. Inhibition of cyclo-oxygenase results in decreased prostaglandin synthesis. The antipyretic action occurs by decreasing prostaglandin synthesis in the hypothalamus resulting in an increase in peripheral blood flow and heat loss, as well as promoting sweating. The mechanism to close patent ductus arteriosus is not known. **Time to peak levels:** 1–2 hr. **Onset:** 30 min for analgesia. **Peak serum levels:** 1–2 hr. **Duration:** 4–6 hr for analgesia. **t½:** 1.8–2 hr. 45–79% excreted in the urine.

SIDE EFFECTS: Ibuprofen: Dizziness, rash, nausea, epigastric/GI pain, heartburn. **Ibuprofen lysine:** Skin lesion/irritation, *SEPSIS*, GI disorders, anemia, *INTRAVENTRICULAR HEMORRHAGE*, impaired renal function, *APNEA*, respiratory failure, RTI.

DOSAGE: OTC: Oral Drops

Antipyretic.

Children, 6–11 months (12–17 pounds): 50 mg (1.25 mL) q 6–8 hr, up to 4 times per day. **12–23 months (18–23 pounds):** 75 mg (1.875 mL) q 6–8 hr, up to 4 times per day.

DOSAGE: OTC: Oral Suspension

Pain, fever.

Children, 2–3 years (24–35 pounds): 100 mg (5 mL) q 6–8 hr, up to 4 times per day. **4–5 years (36–47 pounds):** 150 mg (7.5 mL) q 6–8 hr, up to 4 times per day. **6–8 years (48–59 pounds):** 200 mg (10 mL) q 6–8 hr, up to 4 times per day. **9–10 years (60–71 pounds):** 250 mg (12.5 mL) q 6–8 hr, up to 4 times per day. **11 years (72–95 pounds):** 300 mg (15 mL) q 6–8 hr, up to 4 times per day.

DOSAGE: OTC: Chewable Tablets (50 mg)

Pain, fever.

Children, 4–5 years (36–47 pounds): 150 mg (3 tablets) q 6–8 hr, up to 4 times per day. **6–8 years (48–59 pounds):** 200 mg (4 tablets) q 6–8 hr, up to 4 times per day. **9–10 years (60–71 pounds):** 250 mg (5 tablets) q 6–8 hr, up to 4 times per day. **11 years (72–95 pounds):** 300 mg (6 tablets) q 6–8 hr, up to 4 times per day. Usually use weight to dose; otherwise, use age.

DOSAGE: OTC: Junior Strength Chewable Tablets (100 mg)

Pain, fever.

Children, 6–8 years (48–59 pounds): 200 mg (2 tablets) q 6–8 hr, up to 4 times per day. **9–10 years (60–71 pounds):** 250 mg (2.5 tablets) q 6–8 hr, up to 4 times per day. **11 years (72–95 pounds):** 300 mg (3 tablets) q 6–8 hr, up to 4 times per day. Use weight to dose; otherwise use age.

DOSAGE: IV infusion IBUPROFEN LYSINE

Patent ductus arteriosus.

10 mg/kg by IV infusion over 15 min for one dose and then 5

mg/kg 24 and 48 hr later, with all doses based on birth weight. Administration of the second or third dose to an infant with urinary output less than 0.6 mL/kg/hr should be delayed until renal function returns to normal.

NEED TO KNOW

1. Ibuprofen lysine is contraindicated in preterm infants with a proven or suspected infection not receiving treatment; congenital heart disease needing a patent ductus arteriosus to acheive satisfactory pulmonary or systemic blood flow; thrombocytopenia; in those who are bleeding (especially those with active intracranial hemorrhage or GI bleeding); a coagulation defect, proven or suspected necrotizing enterocolitis, or significant impaired renal function.
2. Ibuprofen lysine may alter the usual signs of infection. Use the drug with extra care in the presence of controlled infection and in infants at risk of infection. Use with caution in infants with elevated total bilirubin.
3. If the ductus arteriosus closes or is significantly reduced in size after completion of the first course of ibuprofen lysine, no further doses are necessary. If during continued treatment the ductus arteriosus fails to close or reopens, then a second course of ibuprofen, alternative pharmacologic therapy, or surgery may be necessary.
4. Do not administer ibuprofen lysine simultaneously in the same IV line with TPN. If necessary, interrupt TPN for 15 min prior to and after drug administration.
5. Children's Chewable Tablets are for children, 4–11 years; Junior Strength Tablets are for children, 6–11 years; Oral Suspension is for children 2–11 years; and, Oral Drops are for children 6 months–3 years.
6. Oral Drops: Consult a provider before giving to children who are less than 6 months of age or weigh less than 24 pounds.
7. Oral Suspension: Consult a provider before giving to children who are less than 2 years or weigh less than 24 pounds.
8. Chewable Tablets (50 mg): Consult a provider before giving to

children who are less than 4 years or weigh less than 36 pounds.

9. Chewable Tablets (100 mg): Consult a provider before giving to children who are less than 6 years or weigh less than 48 pounds.
10. Take with a snack, milk, antacid, or meals to decrease GI upset. Report N&V, diarrhea, or constipation.

Insulin injection (Regular insulin)

(**IN**-sue-lin)

OTC: Human Insulin: Humulin R, Novolin R, Novolin R PenFill, Novolin R Prefilled. **Pork Insulin:** Regular Iletin II.

CLASSIFICATION(S): Insulin product

USES: Suitable for treatment of diabetic coma, diabetic acidosis, or other emergency situations. Especially suitable for the client suffering from labile diabetes.

ACTION/KINETICS: Rarely administered as the sole agent due to its short duration of action. Injections of 100 units/mL are clear; cloudy, colored solutions should not be used. Regular insulin is the only preparation suitable for IV administration. Available only as 100 units/mL. **Onset, SC:** 30–60 min; **IV:** 10–30 min. **Peak, SC:** 2–5 hr; **IV:** 15–30 min. **Duration, SC:** 8–12 hr; **IV:** 30–60 min. Is compatible with all other insulins.

SIDE EFFECTS: Hypoglycemia, hypokalemia, injection site reaction, lipodystrophy, pruritus, rash.

DOSAGE: SC

Diabetes.

Children: 2–4 units. Injection is given 15–30 min before meals and at bedtime.

NEED TO KNOW

1. Report adverse effects or lack of sugar control. Continue diet, exercise, and weight control.

Ipratropium bromide
(eye-prah-**TROH**-pee-um)
Rx: Atrovent, Atrovent HFA.

B

CLASSIFICATION(S): Cholinergic blocking drug
USES: **Nasal spray:** (1) Symptomatic relief (using 0.03%) of rhinorrhea associated with allergic and nonallergic perennial rhinitis in clients over 6 years. (2) Symptomatic relief (using 0.06%) of rhinorrhea associated with the common cold in those aged 5 and older.
ACTION/KINETICS: Antagonizes the action of acetylcholine. Prevents the increase in intracellular levels of cyclic guanosine monophosphate, which is caused by the interaction of acetylcholine with muscarinic receptors in bronchial smooth muscle; this leads to bronchodilation which is primarily a local, site-specific effect. Poorly absorbed into the systemic circulation. **t½, elimination:** 1.6 hr after use of the nasal spray.
SIDE EFFECTS: **Nasal spray:** Headache, pharyngitis, URTI, epistaxis, nasal dryness, nausea, nasal irritation, dry mouth/throat, taste perversion. *BRONCHOSPASM, LARYNGOSPASM, ANAPHYLAXIS.*

DOSAGE: Nasal Spray, 0.03%

Perennial rhinitis.

Children, 6 years and older: 2 sprays (42 mcg) per nostril 2–3 times per day for a total daily dose of 168–252 mcg/day. Optimum dose varies.

DOSAGE: Nasal Spray, 0.06%

Rhinitis due to the common cold.

Children, 12 years and older: 2 sprays (84 mcg) per nostril 3–4 times per day for a total daily dose of 504–672 mcg/day. **5–11 years:** 2 sprays (84 mcg) per nostril 3 times per day (total dose of 504 mcg/day). Safety and efficacy for use for the common cold for more than 4 days have not been determined.

Rhinorrhea associated with seasonal allergic rhinitis.

Children, 5 years and older: 2 sprays (84 mcg) per nostril 4 times per day (total of 672 mcg/day). Safety and efficacy for use beyond 3 weeks have not been determined.

NEED TO KNOW

1. Safety and efficacy of the nasal spray (0.03%) in children less than 6 years of age and of the nasal spray (0.06%) in children less than 5 years of age has not been determined.
2. Take only as directed; shake nasal spray; do not exceed 8 sprays in each nostril in 24 hr.
3. Transient dizziness, insomnia, blurred vision, or excessive weakness may occur, use caution.

Isoproterenol hydrochloride

(eye-so-proe-**TER**-e-nole)

Rx: Isuprel, Isuprel Mistometer.

C

CLASSIFICATION(S): Sympathomimetic

USES: **Inhalation:** Relief of bronchospasms associated with acute and chronic asthma, chronic bronchitis, or emphysema. **Injection:** Bronchospasm during anesthesia.

ACTION/KINETICS: Produces pronounced stimulation of both beta-1 and beta-2 receptors of the heart, bronchi, skeletal muscle vasculature, and the GI tract. Has both positive inotropic and chronotropic activity resulting in increased CO; systolic BP may increase while diastolic BP may decrease. Thus, mean arterial BP may not change or may be decreased. Causes less hyperglycemia than epinephrine, but produces bronchodilation and the same degree of CNS excitation. Readily absorbed after aerosol use. **Inhalation: Onset,** 2–5 min; **peak effect:** 3–5 min; **duration:** 1–3 hr.

SIDE EFFECTS: Nausea, warmth, diaphoresis, dizziness, pallor, visual blurring, shakiness, weakness, headache, dyspnea.

DOSAGE: Inhalation ISOPROTERENOL HYDROCHLORIDE

Acute bronchial asthma.

Children: *Hand bulb nebulizer:* Give 5–15 deep inhalations of the 1:200 solution. *Metered dose inhaler (aerosol):* One inhalation (103 mcg). Wait 1 min to determine effect before considering a second inhalation. Repeat up to 5 times per day, if necessary.

Bronchospasm.

Children: For acute bronchospasms, use the 1:200 solution. Do not use more than 0.25 mL of the 1:200 solution for each 10–15 min programmed treatment.

NEED TO KNOW

1. Administration to children, except where noted, is the same as that for adults; their smaller ventilatory exchange capacity will permit a proportionally smaller aerosol intake. For their acute bronchospasms, use 1:200 solution.
2. In children, no more than 0.25 mL of the 1:200 solution should be used for each 10–15 min of programmed treatment.
3. The initial IV dose of isoproterenol in children (7 to 19 years) ranges between 0.05–0.17 mcg/kg/min, which is increased gradually by 0.1 to 0.2 mcg/kg/min at intervals of 15 to 20 min, titrated to clinical response. The maximum dose range used is 1.3–2.7 mcg/kg/min. General postoperative pediatric cardiac clients with bradycardia require lower doses (0.029 ± 0.002 mcg/kg/min) of IV isoproterenol than do asthma clients (0.5 ± 0.21 mcg/kg/min).
4. Rinse mouth and equipment with water to remove drug residue and minimize dryness after inhalation.
5. Sputum and saliva may appear pink after inhalation therapy; do not become alarmed.
6. Do not use more often than prescribed; overuse can cause se-

vere cardiac and respiratory problems. Report any chest pain/ tightness or increased SOB.

Lamotrigine ■ C

(lah-**MOH**-trih-jeen)

Rx: Lamictal, Lamictal Chewable Dispersible Tablets.

CLASSIFICATION(S): Anticonvulsant, miscellaneous

USES: (1) Adjunct in treatment of partial seizures in children 2 years and older. (2) Adjunct in treating seizures in children 2 years and older with Lennox-Gastaut syndrome. (3) Adjunct to treat primary generalized tonic-clonic seizures in children 2 years and older.

ACTION/KINETICS: May act to inhibit voltage-sensitive sodium channels. This effect stabilizes neuronal membranes and modulates presynaptic transmitter release of excitatory amino acids such as glutamate and aspartate. Rapidly and completely absorbed after PO use with negligible first-pass metabolism; **Peak plasma levels:** 1.4–4.8 hr. The chewable/dispersible tablets are equivalent in terms of rate and extent of absorption whether they are given as dispersed in water, chewed and swallowed, or swallowed whole as compared with compressed tablets. Metabolized by the liver with metabolites and unchanged drug excreted mainly through the urine (94%). Lamotrigine induces its own metabolism following multiple doses. **Plasma protein binding:** About 55%.

SIDE EFFECTS: **When used as adjunctive therapy:** Dizziness, ataxia, somnolence, headache, diplopia, blurred vision, N&V, rash. **When used as monotherapy:** N&V, abnormal coordination, dyspepsia, dizziness, rhinitis, anxiety, insomnia, infection, pain, weight decrease, chest pain, dysmenorrhea.

DOSAGE: Tablets; Tablets, Chewable Dispersible

Partial seizures, lamotrigine added to valproic acid.

Children, over 12 years: Weeks 1 and 2, 25 mg q other day. **Weeks 3 and 4,** 25 mg every day. **Week 5 onwards to maintenance:** Increase by 25–50 mg/day q 1 to 2 weeks. **Maintenance, usual:** 100–400 mg/day in 1 or 2 divided doses (100–200 mg/day with valproate alone). **2–12 years: Weeks 1 and 2,** 0.15 mg/kg/day in 1 or 2 divided doses, rounded down to the nearest whole tablet. **Weeks 3 and 4,** 0.3 mg/kg/day in 1 or 2 divided doses; round down to the nearest whole tablet. **Week 5 onwards to maintenance:** Increase dose q 1 to 2 weeks as follows: Calculate 0.3 mg/kg/day; round this amount down to the nearest whole tablet and add this amount to the previously administered daily dose. **Maintenance, usual:** 1–5 mg/kg/day in 1 or 2 divided doses, not to exceed 200 mg/day. Maintenance doses in children weighing less than 30 kg may need to be increased by as much as 50%, based on clinical response.

If dosage is calculated on a weight basis in children 2–12 years, use the following guide: 6.7 to less than 14 kg: Weeks 1 and 2, 2 mg every other day. **Weeks 3 and 4,** 2 mg per day. **14.1 to less than 27 kg: Weeks 1 and 2,** 2 mg per day. **Weeks 3 and 4,** 4 mg per day. **27.1 to less than 34 kg: Weeks 1 and 2,** 4 mg per day. **Weeks 3 and 4:** 8 mg per day. **34.1 to less than 40 kg: Weeks 1 and 2,** 5 mg per day. **Weeks 3 and 4,** 10 mg per day. Give daily doses using the most appropriate combination of 2 mg and 5 mg tablets. **Maintenance:** 1–3 mg/kg/day (see above).

Partial seizures, clients taking enzyme-inducing antiepileptic drugs (e.g., carbamazepine, phenobarbital, phenytoin, primidone) without valproic acid.

Children, over 12 years: Weeks 1 and 2, 50 mg/day. **Weeks 3 and 4,** 100 mg/day in 2 divided doses. **Week 5 onwards to maintenance:** Increase by 100 mg/day q 1–2 weeks. **Maintenance, usual:** 300–500 mg/day in 2 divided doses. **2–12**

years: Weeks 1 and 2, 0.6 mg/kg/day in 2 divided doses, rounded down to the nearest whole tablet. **Weeks 3 and 4,** 1.2 mg/kg/day in 2 divided doses, rounded down to the nearest whole tablet. **Week 5 onwards to maintenance:** Increase the dose as follows q 1–2 weeks: Calculate 1.2 mg/kg/day and round down to the nearest whole tablet; add this amount to the previously administered daily dose. **Maintenance, usual:** 5–15 mg/kg/day, to a maximum of 400 mg/day in 2 divided doses. Doses for those weighing less than 30 kg may need to be increased by as much as 50%, based on clinical response.

Partial seizures, clients taking antiepileptic drugs other than carbamazepine, phenobarbital, phenytoin, primidone, or valproate.

Children, older than 12 years: Weeks 1 and 2: 25 mg/day; **weeks 3 and 4:** 50 mg/day; **weeks 5 onwards to maintenance:** Increase by 50 mg/day q 1–2 weeks; **maintenance, usual:** 225–375 mg/day in 2 divided doses. **2–12 years: Weeks 1 and 2:** 0.3 mg/kg/day in 1 or 2 divided doses, rounded down to the nearest whole tablet; **Weeks 3 and 4:** 0.6 mg/kg/day in 2 divided doses, rounded down to the nearest whole tablet; **Week 5 onward to maintenance:** Dose should be increased every 1–2 weeks as follows: Calculate 0.6 mg/kg/day and round this amount down to the nearest whole tablet, and add this amount to the previously administered daily dose; **maintenance, usual:** 4.5–7.5 mg/kg/day, up to a maximum of 300 mg/day in 2 divided doses. Maintenance doses in children weighing less than 30 kg may need to be increased by as much as 50%, based on clinical response.

NEED TO KNOW

1. Abrupt withdrawal may increase seizure frequency.
2. Dose based on the therapeutic response since a therapeutic plasma level has not been determined.
3. If decided to discontinue lamotrigine therapy, a stepwise reduction of dose over 2 weeks (about 50% per week) is recom-

mended unless safety concerns mandate a more rapid withdrawal.

4. Swallow chewable dispersible tablets whole, chewed, or dispersed in water or diluted fruit juice. If chewed, drink a small amount of water or diluted fruit juice to help in swallowing. To disperse chewable tablets, add the tablets to 5 mL (or enough to cover the drug) of liquid. About 1 min later, when tablets are completely dispersed, swirl the solution and consume the entire amount immediately. Do not take partial amounts of dispersed tablets.
5. Immediately report loss of seizure control or occurrence of a rash.

Lansoprazole
(lan-**SAHP**-rah-zohl)
Rx: Prevacid, Prevacid IV.

B

CLASSIFICATION(S): Proton pump inhibitor
USES: (1) Short-term treatment (up to 8 weeks) for healing and symptomatic relief of all grades of erosive esophagitis. Maintain healing of erosive esophagitis. (2) Heartburn and other symptoms of GERD. (3) Short-term treatment of symptomatic GERD and erosive esophagitis including in children, aged 1 to 17 years (PO only).
ACTION/KINETICS: Drug is a gastric acid (proton) pump inhibitor in that it blocks the final step of acid production. Suppresses gastric acid secretion by inhibition of the (H^+, K^+)-ATPase system located at the secretory surface of the parietal cells in the stomach. Absorption begins only after lansoprazole granules leave the stomach, but absorption is rapid. **Peak plasma levels:** 1.7 hr. **Mean plasma $t_{1/2}$, PO:** 1.5 hr. Metabolized in the liver with metabolites excreted through both the urine (33%) and feces (66%). **Plasma protein binding:** More than 97%.
SIDE EFFECTS: Diarrhea, headache, N&V, constipation, rash. *GI HEMORRHAGE, RECTAL HEMORRHAGE, PANCREATITIS, PANCYTOPENIA, APLASTIC ANEMIA,*

STEVENS-JOHNSON SYNDROME, TOXIC EPIDERMAL NECROLYSIS, CARCINOMA, ALLERGIC REACTION, ANAPHYLACTOID-LIKE REACTION.

DOSAGE: Capsules, Delayed-Release; Oral Suspension, Delayed-Release; Tablets, Orally Disintegrating, Delayed-Release

GERD.

Children, 12–17 years: 15 mg once daily for up to 8 weeks. **1–11 years, 30 kg or less:** 15 mg/day for up to 12 weeks; if symptoms remain after 2 or more weeks, can increase the dose to 30 mg twice a day. **1–11 years, over 30 kg:** 30 mg/day for up to 12 weeks; if symptoms remain after 2 or more weeks, can increase the dose to 30 mg twice a day.

Erosive esophagitis.

Children, 12–17 years, short-term treatment: 30 mg once daily before meals for up to 8 weeks. **1–11 years, short-term treatment, 30 kg or less:** 15 mg/day for up to 12 weeks; if symptoms remain after 2 or more weeks, can increase the dose to 30 mg twice a day. **1–11 years, short-term treatment, over 30 kg:** 30 mg/day for up to 12 weeks; if symptoms remain after 2 or more weeks, can increase the dose to 30 mg twice a day.

NEED TO KNOW

1. Do not crush or chew any lansoprazole PO product.
2. For those unable to swallow capsules, open delayed-release capsule and sprinkle contents on a tablespoon of applesauce, *Ensure,* pudding, cottage cheese, yogurt, or strained pears and swallow immediately. Alternatively, contents of the capsule can be mixed with about 2 oz of either apple, orange, or tomato juice, mixed briefly, and swallowed immediately.
3. To give capsules with an NG tube in place, open capsule and mix intact granules with 40 mL of apple juice; do not use other liquids. Instill through NG tube into the stomach, flushing with additional apple juice to clear the tube.

4. May have to stop drug if reports of any severe headaches, worsening of symptoms, fever, chills, or diarrhea.
5. Avoid hazardous activities until drug effects realized; dizziness many occur.

Levothyroxine sodium (T_4)

(lee-voh-thigh-**ROX**-een) **A**

Rx: Levothroid, Levoxyl, Synthroid, Thyro-Tabs, Tirosint, Unithroid.

CLASSIFICATION(S): Thyroid product

USES: Replacement or supplemental therapy for congenital or acquired hypothyroidism of any etiology.

ACTION/KINETICS: Levothyroxine is the synthetic sodium salt of the levoisomer of T_4 (tetraiodothyronine). Absorption from the GI tract is incomplete and variable, especially when taken with food. Has a slower onset but a longer duration than sodium liothyronine. **Time to peak therapeutic effect:** 3–4 weeks. **t½:** 6–7 days in a euthyroid person, 9–10 days in a hypothyroid client, and 3–4 days in a hyperthyroid client. **Duration:** 1–3 weeks after withdrawal of chronic therapy. *NOTE:* All levothyroxine products are not bioequivalent; thus, changing brands is not recommended.

SIDE EFFECTS: Symptoms of hyperthyroidism.

DOSAGE: Capsules; Tablets

Congenital hypothyroidism.

Children, 12 years and older: 2–3 mcg/kg once daily until the adult daily dose (usually 150 mcg) is reached. **6–12 years:** 4–5 mcg/kg/day or 100–150 mcg once daily. **1–5 years:** 5–6 mcg/kg/day or 75–100 mcg once daily. **6–12 months of age:** 6–8 mcg/kg/day or 50–75 mcg once daily. **Less than 6 months of age:** 8–10 mcg/kg/day or 25–50 mcg once daily.

DOSAGE: IM; IV

Hypothyroidism.

Children, IV, IM: A dose of 75% of the usual PO pediatric dose should be given.

NEED TO KNOW

1. Errors have occurred when prescribers have ordered 0.25 mg (250 mcg) instead of the correct dose of 0.025 mg (25 mcg). Be careful with decimal point placements and when converting a dose from micrograms to milligrams.
2. Take with a full glass of water to prevent choking, gagging, dysphagia, or getting tablets stuck in the throat.
3. In infants with congenital or acquired hypothyroidism, institute therapy with full doses as soon as the diagnosis is made.
4. In infants and children who cannot swallow tablets, the correct dosage tablet may be crushed and suspended in a small amount of formula or water and given by dropper or spoon. The crushed tablet may also be sprinkled over cooked cereal or applesauce.
5. Note the child's height, weight, and psychomotor development.
6. Take at the same time each day on an empty stomach 1 hr before or 2–3 hr after a meal. Take in the morning to prevent insomnia. Do not take with food unless specifically instructed; may interfere with absorption. Avoid iodine-rich foods.
7. Report severe headache, palpitations, chest pain, diarrhea, irritability, excitability, insomnia, intolerance to heat, significant weight loss, and/or excessive sweating.
8. Child may experience hair loss; should regrow. Return for evaluation of bone age, growth, labs, and psychomotor functioning.

Lisinopril

(lie-**SIN**-oh-prill)

Rx: Prinivil, Zestril.

C

CLASSIFICATION(S): Antihypertensive, ACE inhibitor

USES: Hypertension in children, aged 6–16 years.

ACTION/KINETICS: Inhibits angiotensin-converting enzyme resulting in decreased plasma angiotensin II, which leads to decreased vasopressor activity and decreased aldosterone secretion. Both supine and standing BPs are reduced. Only 25% of a PO dose is absorbed. **Onset:** 1 hr. **Peak serum levels:** 7 hr. **Duration:** 24 hr. **$t\frac{1}{2}$:** 12 hr. 100% of the drug is excreted unchanged in the urine.

SIDE EFFECTS: Chest pain, dizziness, headache, hypotension, fatigue, diarrhea, URTI.

DOSAGE: Tablets

Essential hypertension, used alone.

Children, over 6 years, initial: 0.07 mg/kg once daily (up to 5 mg total). Adjust dose according to BP response; doses above 0.61 mg/kg (or in excess of 40 mg) have not been studied in children.

NEED TO KNOW

1. Do not use in children less than 6 years or in children with a GFR less than 30 mL/min/1.73 m^2.
2. Maximum antihypertensive effects may not be observed for 2–4 weeks.
3. Avoid all potassium supplements as well as foods high in potassium, unless otherwise directed.
4. Report new or unusual side effects or aggravation of existing conditions, as well as sore throat, hoarseness, cough, chest pain, difficulty breathing, or swelling of hands, feet, or face.

Loperamide hydrochloride

B

(loh-**PER**-ah-myd)

OTC: Diar-aid Caplets, Imodium, Imodium A-D Caplets, K-Pek II, Kaopectate II Caplets, Maalox Anti-Diarrheal Caplets, Neo-Diaral, Pepto Diarrhea Control. **Rx:** Imodium.

CLASSIFICATION(S): Antidiarrheal

USES: Rx: (1) Symptomatic relief of acute nonspecific diarrhea and of chronic diarrhea associated with inflammatory bowel disease. **OTC:** Control symptoms of diarrhea, including traveler's diarrhea.

ACTION/KINETICS: Slows intestinal motility by acting on the nerve endings and/or intramural ganglia embedded in the intestinal wall. The prolonged retention of the feces in the intestine results in reducing the volume of the stools, increasing viscosity, and decreasing fluid and electrolyte loss. **Time to peak effect, capsules:** 5 hr; **PO solution:** 2.5 hr. **$t_{1/2}$:** 9.1–14.4 hr. Twenty-five percent excreted unchanged in the feces.

SIDE EFFECTS: Abdominal pain/distention/discomfort, constipation, dry mouth, N&V, epigastric distress, dizziness, drowsiness.

DOSAGE: Rx: Capsules

Acute diarrhea.

Children: *Day 1 doses:* **8–12 years:** 2 mg 3 times per day; **6–8 years:** 2 mg twice a day; **2–5 years:** 1 mg 3 times per day using only the liquid. *After day 1:* 1 mg/10 kg after a loose stool (total daily dosage should not exceed day 1 recommended doses).

DOSAGE: OTC: Capsules, Liquid, Tablets

Acute diarrhea.

Children, 9–11 years: 2 mg after the first LBM followed by 1 mg after each subsequent LBM, not to exceed 6 mg/day for no more than 2 days. **6–8 years:** 1 mg after the first bowel movement followed by 1 mg after each subsequent LBM, not to exceed 4 mg/day for no more than 2 days.

NEED TO KNOW

1. Safe use in children under 2 years has not been established.
2. Children under 3 years are more sensitive to the narcotic effects of loperamide.
3. May cause a dry mouth; try ice, sugarless gum, and candy to alleviate.
4. OTC products are not intended for use in children less than 6 years unless provider prescribed.
5. In *acute diarrhea,* discontinue after 48 hr and report if ineffective.
6. In children, dietary treatment of diarrhea is preferred. Avoid apple juices, formulas, and high fat or spicy foods.

Loratidine

(loh-**RAH**-tih-deen) **B**

OTC: Oral Solution: Claritin Allergy Children's, Clear-Atadine Children's. **Syrup:** Alavert Children's, Children's Loratidine Syrup, Claritin, Dimetapp Children's ND Non-Drowsy Allergy, Non-Drowsy Allergy Relief for Kids. **Tablets, Chewable:** Claritin Children's Allergy. **Tablets, Orally Disintegrating:** Alavert, Claritin RediTabs, Dimetapp Children's ND Non-Drowsy Allergy, Non-Drowsy Allergy Relief, Triaminic Allerchews.

CLASSIFICATION(S): Antihistamine, second generation, piperidine

USES: (1) Relief of nasal and nonnasal symptoms of seasonal allergic rhinitis, including runny nose, itchy and watery eyes, itchy palate, and sneezing. (2) Relief of itching due to hives in children 6 years and older.

ACTION/KINETICS: Metabolized in the liver to active metabolite descarboethoxyloratidine. Low to no sedative and anticholinergic effects; no antiemetic effect. **Onset:** 1–3 hr. **Maximum effect:** 8–12 hr. Food delays absorption. **t½, loratidine:** 8.4 hr; **t½, descar-**

boethoxyloratidine: 28 hr. **Duration:** 24 hr. Excreted through both the urine and feces.

SIDE EFFECTS: Headache, somnolence, fatigue, dry mouth.

DOSAGE: Oral Solution; Syrup; Tablets; Tablets, Oral Disintegrating; Tablets, Rapidly Disintegrating

Allergic rhinitis, chronic idiopathic urticaria.

Children, 6 years and older: 10 mg once daily. **In children 6 years and older with impaired kidney function (GFR <30 mL/min):** 10 mg every other day initially.

NEED TO KNOW

1. Do not use in children less than 6 years.
2. Use the syrup or chewable/orally disintegrating tablets for children ages 6 to 11.
3. Use caution. The concentration of the syrup is 5 mg/5 mL.
4. Take on an empty stomach; food may delay absorption. If stomach upset occurs, can take with food.
5. If using rapidly disintegrating tablets, place under the tongue. Disintegration occurs within seconds, after which the tablet contents may be swallowed with or without water.
6. Avoid prolonged or excessive exposure to direct or artificial sunlight.

Mebendazole
(meh-**BEN**-dah-zohl)
Rx: Vermox.

C

CLASSIFICATION(S): Anthelmintic
USES: Single or mixed infections of whipworm, pinworm, roundworm, and common and American hookworm. Not effective for hydatid disease.
ACTION/KINETICS: Anthelmintic effect occurs by blocking the glucose uptake of the organisms, thereby reducing their energy until death results. It also inhibits the formation of microtubules in the helminth. **Peak plasma levels:** 2–4 hr. Poorly absorbed from the GI tract. Excreted in feces as unchanged drug or metabolites.
SIDE EFFECTS: Transient abdominal pain, diarrhea.

DOSAGE: Tablets, Chewable

Whipworm, roundworm, and hookworm.

Children: 1 tablet morning and evening on 3 consecutive days.

Pinworms.

1 tablet, one time. All treatments can be repeated after 3 weeks if the client is not cured.

NEED TO KNOW

1. Use with caution in children under 2 years.
2. Tablets may be chewed, swallowed, or crushed and mixed with food. Fasting or purging are not required.
3. Immobilization followed by death of parasites is slow. Complete clearance from the GI tract may take up to 3 days after initiation of treatment.
4. Report if S&S do not improve or worsen after 3 weeks.

Meloxicam ■ C

(meh-**LOX**-ih-kam)

Rx: Mobic.

CLASSIFICATION(S): Nonsteroidal anti-inflammatory

USES: Relief of signs and symptoms of pauciarticular or polyarticular course juvenile rheumatoid arthritis in clients 2 years and older.

ACTION/KINETICS: Anti-inflammatory effect is likely due to inhibition of cyclo-oxygenase. Inhibition of cyclo-oxygenase results in decreased prostaglandin synthesis. Effective in reducing joint swelling, pain, and morning stiffness, as well as to increase mobility in those with inflammatory disease. Does not alter the course of the disease, however. Prolonged drug absorption. Steady state reached in 5 days. Metabolized in the liver by P450-mediated metabolism. **Peak:** 4–5 hr. **$t_{1/2}$, elimination:** 15–20 hr. Excreted in about equal amounts in the urine and feces.

SIDE EFFECTS: Headache, dizziness, insomnia, rash, abdominal pain/cramps, diarrhea, N&V, constipation, flatulence, dyspepsia/indigestion, UTI, edema, URTI, pharyngitis.

DOSAGE: Oral Suspension Tablets

Pauciarticular/polyarticular course juvenile rhematoid arthritis.

Recommended PO dose: 0.125 mg/kg once daily, up to a maximum of 7.5 mg daily. The following dosage recommendations are based on weight using the oral suspension (1.5 mg/mL): **12 kg (26 lbs):** 1 mL (1.5 mg); **24 kg (54 lbs):** 2 mL (3 mg); **36 kg (80 lbs):** 3 mL (4.5 mg); **48 kg (106 lbs):** 4 mL (6 mg); **greater or equal to 60 kg (132 lbs):** 5 mL (7.5 mg).

NEED TO KNOW

1. Do not use in those who have exhibited asthma, urticaria, or allergic-type reactions after taking aspirin or other NSAIDs (anaphylaxis is possible).
2. Use the lowest dose for the shortest duration consistent with

individual client treatment goals. Adjust dose to suit the individual client's needs.

3. The oral suspension, 7.5 mg/5 mL or 15 mg/10 mL, may be substituted for meloxicam tablets, 7.5 or 15 mg respectively.
4. May be taken without regard to meals.
5. Shake the oral suspension gently before using.
6. Report unusual or persistent side effects including dyspepsia, abdominal pain, dizziness, and changes in stool or skin color.

Methylphenidate hydrochloride ■ C

(meth-ill-**FEN**-ih-dayt)

Rx: Capsules, Extended-Release: Metadate CD, Ritalin LA. **Oral Solution**: Methylin. **Tablets**: Methylin, Ritalin. **Tablets, Chewable**: Methylin. **Tablets, Extended-Release**: Concerta, Metadate ER, Methylin ER, Ritalin-SR. **Transdermal Patch**: Daytrana, **C-II.**

CLASSIFICATION(S): CNS stimulant

USES: Attention-deficit disorders (ADD) and attention-deficit/hyperactivity disorders (ADHD) in children as part of overall treatment regimen. Syndrome characterized by moderate to severe distractibility, short attention span, hyperactivity, emotional lability, and impulsivity. Transdermal patch used only for ADHD.

ACTION/KINETICS: May activate the brain stem arousal system and cortex to produce stimulation. In children with ADD, methylphenidate causes decreases in motor restlessness with an increased attention span. Rapidly and well absorbed from the GI tract. Food delays peak levels of the chewable tablets by about 1 hr. **Peak blood levels, children:** 1.9 hr for tablets; 1–2 hr for chewable tablets; and, 4.7 hr for extended-release tablets. **Duration:** 4–6 hr. **t½ tablets, chewable tablets, Concerta tablets:** 1–3.5 hr; **t½**, Metatate CD: 6.8 hr. Metabolized by the liver and excreted by the kidney. *NOTE:* The various methylphenidate products have different pharmacokinetic properties.

SIDE EFFECTS: Headache, URTI, abdominal pain, anorexia, insomnia, vomiting, accidental injury, nervousness, anxiety/irritability, rhinitis, fever, loss of appetite, weight loss during chronic use, tachycardia.

DOSAGE: Capsules, Extended-Release; Oral Solution; Tablets, Chewable; Tablets, Immediate-Release; Tablets, Extended-Release

Attention-deficit/hyperactivity disorder.

Individualize dose. Children, 6 years and older, initial: 5 mg twice a day before breakfast and lunch; **then,** increase gradually by 5–10 mg/week to a maximum of 60 mg/day. If no improvement is noted after a 1-month period, discontinue the drug.

DOSAGE: Transdermal Patch

Attention-deficit/hyperactivity disorder.

Children, 6–12 years, initial: 10 mg over 9 hr for the first week with the patch applied to the client's hip 2 hr before an effect is needed; remove after 9 hr. **Week 2:** 15 mg over 9 hr; **week 3:** 20 mg over 9 hr; **week 4 and thereafter:** 30 mg over 9 hr.

NEED TO KNOW

1. Do not use concurrent treatment of Concerta, Metadate CD, Ritalin, Ritalin LA, and Ritalin-SR with monoamine oxidase inhibitors and within a minimum of 14 days after stopping MAOI therapy (hypertensive crisis may occur).
2. Do not use in children less than 6 years.
3. Discontinue periodically to assess condition as drug therapy is not indefinite; discontinue at puberty.
4. With ADD, take before breakfast and lunch to avoid interference with sleep. Take Ritalin SR and Concerta tablets whole; do not chew or crush. May swallow whole or sprinkle contents of Metadate CD onto a small amount of applesauce and take immediately. May notice the shell of the Concerta tablet in the stool.

5. Record weight 2 times per week; report any significant loss as this may occur.
6. Report changes in mood, attention span; seizure disorder.
7. Therapy may be interrupted every few months ('drug holiday') to determine if still needed in those responsive to therapy.
8. Children should take the chewable tablets with at least 8 ounces of water or other fluid. Failure to do so may cause choking.

Metoclopramide B
(meh-toe-kloh-**PRAH**-myd)
Rx: Maxolon, Reglan.

CLASSIFICATION(S): Gastrointestinal stimulant
USES: **Parenteral:** (1) Prevention of N&V associated with emetogenic cancer chemotherapy. (2) Stimulate gastric emptying and intestinal transit of barium in clients where delayed emptying interferes with radiological examination of the stomach or small intestine.
ACTION/KINETICS: Dopamine antagonist that acts by increasing sensitivity to acetylcholine; results in increased motility of the upper GI tract and relaxation of the pyloric sphincter and duodenal bulb. Facilitates intubation of the small bowel and speeds transit of a barium meal. **Onset, IV:** 1–3 min; **IM:** 10–15 min; **PO:** 30–60 min. **Duration:** 1–2 hr. **t½:** 5–6 hr. Significant first-pass effect following PO use; unchanged drug and metabolites excreted in urine.
SIDE EFFECTS: Extrapyramidal symptoms, restlessness, drowsiness, fatigue, lassitude, akathisia, dizziness, nausea, diarrhea.

DOSAGE: IM; IV
Prophylaxis of vomiting due to chemotherapy.
Initial: 2 mg/kg IV (1 mg/kg may be adequate for less emetogenic regimens) q 2 hr for two doses, with the first dose 30

min before chemotherapy; **then,** 10 mg or more q 3 hr for three doses. Inject slowly IV over 15 min.

Facilitate small bowel intubation.

IV. Children, 6–14 years: 2.5–5 mg; **less than 6 years:** 0.1 mg/kg. Give a single undiluted dose slowly IV over 1–2 min.

NEED TO KNOW

1. Extrapyramidal effects are more likely to occur in children.
2. Inject slowly IV over 1–2 min to prevent transient feelings of anxiety/restlessness.
3. Drug increases the movements or contractions of the stomach and intestines.
4. Extrapyramidal effects (trembling hands, facial grimacing) should be reported; may be treated with parenteral diphenhydramine.

Mometasone furoate monohydrate

(moh-**MET**-ah-sohn)

C

Rx: Nasonex.

Mometasone furoate

Rx: Powder for Inhalation: Asmanex Twisthaler.

CLASSIFICATION(S): Glucocorticoid

USES: **Mometasone furoate monohydrate. Spray:** (1) Treatment of the nasal symptoms of seasonal allergic rhinitis and perennial allergic rhinitis in children 2 years and older. (2) Prophylaxis of nasal symptoms of seasonal or perennial allergic rhinitis in adolescents 12 years and older. **Mometasone furoate. Powder for Inhalation:** (1) Maintenance treatment of chronic asthma in clients 12 years and older. (2) For clients with asthma who require PO corticosteroid therapy, where adding mometasone may reduce or eliminate the need for PO corticosteroids.

ACTION/KINETICS: Anti-inflammatory due to ability to inhibit prostaglandin synthesis. Also inhibits accumulation of macrophages and leukocytes at sites of inflammation as well as inhibits phagocytosis and lysosomal enzyme release. Metabolized in the liver by CYP3A4 enzymes. **t½:** 5.8 hr. Excreted in the feces and urine. **Plasma protein binding:** 98–99%.

SIDE EFFECTS: For Asmanex: Dry/irritated throat, hoarseness, cough, dry mouth, taste alteration. **For Nasonex:** Headache, pharyngitis, epistaxis, nasal burning/irritation.

DOSAGE: Nasal Spray MOMETASONE FUROATE MONOHYDRATE

Prophylaxis and treatment of seasonal/perennial allergic rhinitis.

Children, over 12 years: 2 sprays (50 mcg in each spray) in each nostril once daily (i.e., total daily dose: 200 mcg). In those with a known seasonal allergen that precipitates seasonal allergic rhinitis, give prophylactically, 200 mcg/day, 2 to 4 weeks prior to the anticipated start of the pollen season. **2–11 years:** One spray (50 mcg) in each nostril once daily (total daily dose: 100 mcg).

DOSAGE: Powder for Inhalation

Chronic asthma.

Recommended starting dose, previous therapy of bronchodilators alone or inhaled corticosteroids: 220 mcg once daily in the evening; **highest recommended daily dose:** 440 mcg. **Recommended starting dose, previous therapy of oral corticosteroids:** 440 mcg twice daily; **highest recommended daily dose:** 880 mcg.

NEED TO KNOW

1. Not indicated to relieve acute bronchospasms.
2. Safety and efficacy of Nasonex has not been determined in children less than 2 years for use in allergic rhinitis and in children less than 18 years to treat nasal polyps.
3. Improvement is usually seen within 11 hours to 2 days after the first dose. Maximum benefit: Within 1 to 2 weeks.
4. The pump may be stored, unused, for up to 1 week without

repriming. If more than 1 week has elapsed between use, reprime by actuating 2 times, or until a fine spray appears.

5. Use regularly as directed. Do not increase dose/frequency; does not increase effectiveness. A spacer facilitates oral inhaler administration.
6. When using oral inhaler, inhale deeply and rapidly and hold breath for about 10 seconds, or as long as possible. Do not breathe out through the inhaler. Rinse mouth/equipment after inhalation use.

Montelukast sodium
(mon-teh-**LOO**-kast)
Rx: Singulair.

B

CLASSIFICATION(S): Antiasthmatic, leukotriene receptor antagonist

USES: (1) Prophylaxis and chronic treatment of asthma in children 12 months of age and older. (2) Relief of symptoms of seasonal allergic rhinitis in children 2 years and older. (3) Relief of symptoms of perennial allergic rhinitis in children 6 months of age and older. (4) Prevention of exercise-induced bronchoconstriction in clients 15 years and older.

ACTION/KINETICS: Cysteinyl leukotrienes and leukotriene receptor occupation are associated with symptoms of asthma, including airway edema, smooth muscle contraction, and inflammation. Montelukast binds with cysteinyl leukotriene receptors thus preventing the action of cysteinyl leukotrienes. Rapidly absorbed after PO use. **Time to peak levels:** 3–4 hr for 10 mg tablet, 2–2.5 hr for 5 mg tablet, and 2 hr for the 4 mg chewable tablet. The 4 mg oral granule formulation is bioequivalent to the 4 mg chewable tablet. Metabolized extensively in the liver by cytochromes CYP3A4 and CYP2C9; mainly excreted in feces. **t½:** 2.7–5.5 hr for healthy, young adults. **Plasma protein binding:** More than 99%.

SIDE EFFECTS: Depend on age of client. Common side effects include headache, nausea, diarrhea, otitis media, rash, pharygitis, sinusitis.

DOSAGE: Granules; Tablets, Chewable

Asthma, Seasonal/perennial allergic rhinitis.

Children, 6 to 14 years: One 5 mg chewable tablet once daily (in the evening for asthma; anytime for allergic rhinitis). **2 to 5 years:** One 4 mg chewable tablet or one 4 mg oral granule packet taken once daily (in the evening for asthma; anytime for allergic rhinitis).

DOSAGE: Granules

Asthma.

Children, 12–23 months: One packet of 4 mg granules once daily in the evening.

Perennial allergic rhinits.

Children, 6–23 months: 1 packet of 4 mg daily.

NEED TO KNOW

1. Do not use to reverse bronchospasm in acute asthma attacks, including status asthmaticus.
2. Safety and efficacy in children less than 12 months of age with asthma, 2 years and younger with seasonal allergic rhinitis, 6 months of age with perennial allergic rhinitis, or 15 years and younger with exercise-induced bronchoconstriction have not been determined.
3. Take daily as prescribed, even when symptom free. Contact provider if asthma is not well controlled.
4. Do not abruptly substitute montelukast for inhaled or oral corticosteroids.
5. Continue drug during acute attacks as well as during symptom free periods.
6. Use short-acting prescribed β-agonist inhalers to treat acute asthma attacks. Report if increased use/frequency of inhalers needed for symptom control.

Nedocromil sodium

(neh-**DAH**-kroh-mill)

Rx: Alocril, Tilade.

B

CLASSIFICATION(S): Antiasthmatic

USES: **Systemic.** Maintenance therapy in children (6 years and older) with mild to moderate bronchial asthma. **Ophthalmic.** Itching associated with allergic conjunctivitis in children over 3 years of age.

ACTION/KINETICS: Is a mast cell stabilizer. Thus, inhibits the release of various mediators, such as histamine, leukotriene C_4, and prostaglandin D_2, from a variety of cell types associated with asthma. **t½:** 3.3 hr. Excreted unchanged. **Plasma protein binding:** About 89%.

SIDE EFFECTS: **After systemic use:** Coughing, bronchospasm, unpleasant taste, pharyngitis, rhinitis, URTI, headache. *BRONCHOSPASM, ANAPHYLAXIS.* **After ophthalmic use:** Headache, nasal congestion, ocular burning/irritation/stinging, unpleasant taste.

DOSAGE: Metered Dose Inhaler

Bronchial asthma.

Children, over 12 years: Two inhalations 4 times per day at regular intervals in order to provide 14 mg/day. If client is under good control on 4 times per day dosing (i.e., requiring inhaled or oral beta agonist no more than twice a week, or no worsening of symptoms occurs with respiratory infections), a lower dose can be tried. In such instances reduce the dose to 10.5 mg/day (i.e., used 3 times per day). Then, after several weeks with good control, the dose can be reduced to 7 mg/day (i.e., used twice a day).

DOSAGE: Ophthalmic Solution

Allergic conjunctivitis.

1 or 2 gtt in each eye twice a day. Continue treatment until

pollen season is over or until exposure to allergen is terminated.

NEED TO KNOW

1. Safety and efficacy have not been established in children less than 6 years.
2. Each actuation releases 1.75 mg.
3. Must be used regularly, even during symptom-free period, in order to achieve beneficial effects.
4. Use eye solution as directed throughout pollen season. Report adverse effects/lack of response.
5. Do not stop inhaler therapy during symptom-free periods; must be taken at regular intervals. Continue to use with other prescribed therapies.
6. Report any persistent headaches, unpleasant taste in mouth that interferes with nutrition, severe nausea, or chest pain. If any coughing, wheezing, or bronchospasm is noted following use, stop drug and report.

Nitazoxanide **B**

(**nye**-tah-**ZOX**-ah-nyde)

Rx: Alinia.

CLASSIFICATION(S): Antiprotozoal

USES: (1) Diarrhea due to *Giardia lamblia* in clients 12 years and older (tablets) and children 1–11 years (PO suspension). (2) Diarrhea due to *Cryptosporidium parvum* in clients 1–11 years and for those 12 years and older who are not infected with HIV.

ACTION/KINETICS: Action is due to interference with the pyruvate: feredoxin oxidoreductase enzyme-dependent electron transfer reaction which is required for anaerobic energy metabolism. Rapidly metabolized to the active tizoxanide and tizoxanide glucuronide. **Maximum plasma levels, active metabolites:** 1–4 hr. Food increases the AUC of both the tablets and suspension. Ex-

creted in the urine, bile, and feces. **Plasma protein binding:** Tizoxanide (active metabolite): more than 99%.
SIDE EFFECTS: Abdominal pain, diarrhea, N&V, headache.

DOSAGE: Oral Suspension; Tablets, Film-Coated

Diarrhea due to Giardia lamblia.

Children, 1–3 years: 5 mL (100 mg) of the oral suspension q 12 hr with food for 3 days. **4–11 years:** 10 mL (200 mg) of the oral suspension q 12 hr with food for 3 days. **Over 12 years:** 1 tablet (500 mg) or 25 mL (500 mg) of the oral suspension q 12 hr with food for 3 days.

Diarrhea due to C. parvum.

Children, 1–3 years: 5 mL (100 mg) of the oral suspension q 12 hr with food for 3 days. **4–11 years:** 10 mL (200 mg) of the oral suspension q 12 hr with food for 3 days. **Over 12 years:** 1 tablet (500 mg) q 12 hr with food for 3 days.

NEED TO KNOW

1. Safety and efficacy of the oral suspension have not been determined in children less than 1 year of age, in children greater than 11 years, or in those with immunodeficiency.
2. After reconstitution, keep bottle tightly closed and shake well before each use. Suspension may be stored for 7 days; discard any unused portion after this period.
3. Confirm flagellate in children. Cysts or trophozites are evident in the stools. Flagellate may cause explosive diarrhea and abdominal cramps. In immunocompromised child who becomes malnourished, response rate may be impaired or death may ensue.
4. Shake well before each use. Administer with food. Inform diabetic clients and caregivers that oral suspension contains 1.48 grams of sucrose/5 mL.
5. May experience GI upset: N&V, abdominal pain, headaches, and diarrhea. Also may discolor urine and give eyes a pale yel-

low discoloration. Report any lack of response, bloody stools, or worsening of S&S.

6. Prevent dehydration, ensure adequate hydration and fluid replacement to compensate for fluid loss through liquid stools.

Nitrofurantoin **B**
(**nye**-troh-fyour-**AN**-toyn)
Rx: Capsules (as macrocrystals): Macrodantin. **Capsules (as monohydrate/macrocrystals)**: Macrobid. **Oral Suspension**: Furadantin.

CLASSIFICATION(S): Urinary anti-infective
USES: UTIs due to susceptible strains of *Escherichia coli, Staphylococcus aureus,* Enterococci, and certain strains of *Enterobacter* and *Klebsiella.*
ACTION/KINETICS: Nitrofurantoin is reduced by bacterial flavoproteins to reactive intermediates that inactivate or alter bacterial ribosomal proteins and other macromolecules. As a result, vital biochemical processes of protein synthesis, aerobic energy metabolism, DNA and RNA synthesis, and cell wall synthesis are inhibited. Is bactericidal in urine at therapeutic doses. Absorption of macrocrystals is slower when compared with the oral suspension (which is readily absorbed from the GI tract). **t½:** 20 min **Urine levels:** 50–250 mcg/mL. The oral suspension is rapidly excreted in urine while excretion of macrocrystals and the monohydrate/macrocrystals is somewhat less.
SIDE EFFECTS: Headache, dizziness, N&V, anorexia, diarrhea, drowsiness, rust-colored or brownish urine. *PANCREATITIS, HEPATIC NECROSIS, STEVENS-JOHNSON SYNDROME, APLASTIC ANEMIA* (rare).

DOSAGE: Capsules (macrocrystals), Oral Suspension
UTIs.

Children, 1 month of age and older: 5–7 mg/kg/day given in 4 divided doses. The following dosages in children, using the oral suspension, are based on average weight in each range receiving 5–6 mg/kg/day given in 4 divided doses: **7–11 kg (15–26 lb):** 2.5 mL 4 times per day; **12–21 kg (27–46 lb):** 5 mL 4 times per day; **22–30 kg (47–68 lb):** 7.5 mL 4 times per day; **31–41 kg (69–91 lb):** 10 mL 4 times per day.

Long-term suppressive therapy.

Children: 1 mg/kg per day, given in a single dose or in 2 divided doses, may be adequate.

DOSAGE: Capsules (monohydrate/macrocrystals)

Uncomplicated UTIs (cystitis).

Children, 1 month of age and over: 5–7 mg/kg/day in 4 equal doses.

NEED TO KNOW

1. Do not use in infants less than 1 month of age.
2. Safety and efficacy of the monohydrate/macrocrystals in children less than 12 years have not been determined.
3. Continue therapy for UTIs for 1 week or for at least 3 days after urine sterility obtained.
4. Do not crush or chew tablets; swallow whole.
5. Take with food or milk to minimize gastric irritation and enhance absorption; complete full course of therapy to prevent bacterial resistance. Avoid alcohol.
6. Acidic foods (prunes, cranberry juice, plums) enhance drug action whereas alkaline foods (milk products) minimize drug action.
7. Report persistent/bothersome side effects or lack of response. May cause dizziness or drowsiness. Breathing problems require immediate help.
8. Any numbness and tingling of extremities or flu-like symptoms must be reported.
9. Report persistent N&V, diarrhea; may be symptoms of a GI superinfection.

Nystatin

(nye-**STAT**-in)

C

Rx: Lozenges: Mycostatin Pastilles. **Oral Suspension**: Mycostatin, Nilstat, Nystex. **Tablets**: Mycostatin. **Topical Cream/Ointment**: Mycostatin, Nilstat, Nystex. **Topical Powder**: Mycostatin, Nystop, Pedi-Dri.

CLASSIFICATION(S): Antifungal

USES: *Candida* infections of the skin, mucous membranes, GI tract, vagina, and mouth (thrush). The drug is too toxic for systemic infections although it can be given PO for intestinal moniliasis infections, as it is not absorbed from the GI tract.

ACTION/KINETICS: Binds to fungal cell membranes (sterols), resulting in altered cellular permeability and leakage of potassium and other essential intracellular components. Is both fungistatic and fungicidal against all species of *Candida*. Poorly absorbed from the GI tract.

SIDE EFFECTS: GI upset, N&V, diarrhea, rash. Nystatin has few toxic effects.

DOSAGE: Lozenges; Oral Suspension; Tablets, Oral

Intestinal candidiasis.

Tablets, 500,000–1,000,000 units 3 times per day; continue treatment for 48 hr after cure to prevent relapse.

Oral candidiasis.

Oral Suspension, children: 400,000–600,000 units 4 times per day (½ dose in each side of mouth, held as long as possible before swallowing); **infants:** 200,000 units 4 times per day; **premature or low birth weight infants:** 100,000 units 4 times per day. **Lozenge, children:** 200,000–400,000 units 4–5 times per day, up to 14 days. *NOTE:* Lozenges should not be chewed or swallowed.

DOSAGE: Topical Cream; Topical Ointment; Topical Powder

Cutaneous or mucocutaneous Candida *infections.*

Apply to affected areas 2–3 times per day, or as indicated, until healing is complete.

NEED TO KNOW

1. Do not use lozenges in children less than 5 years.
2. Do not mix oral suspension in foods; inactivates drug. Remove food from mouth. Drop 1 mL of oral suspension in each side of mouth or apply with a swab to treat oral moniliasis. Swish around and keep in the mouth as long as possible before swallowing.
3. For pediatric use, 250,000 units of cherry flavor nystatin has been frozen in the form of popsicles. If unavailable may swab suspension on oral mucosa.
4. Apply cream or ointment to mycotic lesions with a swab or wear gloves to avoid direct contact with hands; contact dermatitis may ensue.

Omeprazole

(oh-**MEH**-prah-zohl)

OTC: Prilosec OTC. **Rx:** Prilosec.

C

CLASSIFICATION(S): Proton pump inhibitor

USES: Treatment of heartburn and other symptoms associated with GERD.

ACTION/KINETICS: Thought to be a gastric pump inhibitor in that it blocks the final step of acid production by inhibiting the H^+/K^+ ATPase system at the secretory surface of the gastric parietal cell. Both basal and stimulated acid secretions are inhibited. Absorption is rapid. **Peak plasma levels:** 0.5–3.5 hr. **Onset:** Within 1 hr. **$t_{1/2}$:** 0.5–1 hr. **Duration:** Up to 72 hr (due to prolonged binding of the drug to the parietal H^+/K^+ ATPase enzyme). Metabolized in the liver and inactive metabolites are excreted through the urine.

SIDE EFFECTS: Headache, abdominal pain, diarrhea, N&V, URTI, dizziness, rash. *PANCREATITIS, ANAPHYLAXIS* (rare).

DOSAGE:

GERD without esophageal lesions.

Children: For treatment of GERD or other acid-related disorders in children 2 years and older: Give 10 mg for clients weighing less than 20 kg and 20 mg for clients weighing 20 kg or more. Note: On a per kg basis, the doses of omeprazole needed to heal erosive esophagitis are greater for children than for adults.

NEED TO KNOW

1. Efficacy for more than 8 weeks has not been determined. However, if a client does not respond to 8 weeks of therapy, an additional 4 weeks may help.
2. Take capsule at least 1 hr before eating and swallow whole; do not open, chew, or crush. Antacids can be administered with omeprazole.
3. For those who have difficulty swallowing capsules, add 1 tablespoon of applesauce to an empty bowl. Open omeprazole capsule and empty pellets onto applesauce. Mix pellets with the applesauce and swallow immediately. Do not heat or chew the applesauce and do not chew or crush the pellets. Do not store mixture for future use.
4. Take oral suspension on an empty stomach at least 1 hr before a meal.
5. Avoid activities that require mental alertness until drug effects are realized; may cause dizziness.

Ondansetron hydrochloride **B**

(on-**DAN**-sih-tron)

Rx: Zofran, Zofran ODT.

CLASSIFICATION(S): Antiemetic

USES: **Oral:** (1) Prevent N&V resulting from initial and repeated courses of cancer chemotherapy. (2) Prevent N&V associated with initial and repeat courses of moderately emetogenic cancer chemotherapy. **Parenteral:** (1) Prevent N&V associated with initial and repeat courses of emetogenic cancer chemotherapy. (2) Prevention of N&V postoperatively for those in whom nausea and/or vomiting must be avoided, even when the incidence of postoperative N&V is low.

ACTION/KINETICS: Cytotoxic chemotherapy is thought to release serotonin from enterochromaffin cells of the small intestine. The released serotonin may stimulate the vagal afferent nerves through the 5-HT_3 receptors, thus stimulating the vomiting reflex. Ondansetron, a 5-HT_3 antagonist, blocks this effect of serotonin. **Time to peak plasma levels, after PO:** 1.7–2.1 hr. **$t^{1/2}$, after IV use:** 3.5–4.7 hr; **after PO use:** 3.1–6.2 hr, depending on the age. Clients less than 15 years show a shortened plasma half-life after IV use (2.4 hr). Significantly metabolized with 5% of a dose excreted unchanged in the urine.

SIDE EFFECTS: Diarrhea, headache, dizziness, malaise/fatigue, constipation, bradycardia, hypotension, drowsiness/sedation, anxiety/agitation, gynecological disorder, urinary retention, hypoxia, pruritus, pyrexia, shivers.

DOSAGE: IM; IV

Prevention of N&V due to chemotherapy.

Children, 6 months–18 years: Three 0.15 mg/kg doses. The first dose is infused over 15 min starting 30 min before the start of chemotherapy; the second and third doses are given 4 hr and 8 hr, respectively, after the first dose.

Prevent postoperative N&V.

Children, 1 month–12 years, less than 40 kg: 0.1 mg/kg IV over 2–5 min, but not less than 30 seconds. **2–12 years, weighing over 40 kg:** 4 mg IV over 2–5 min, but not less than 30 seconds. For children, give immediately prior to or following anesthesia induction, or postoperatively as needed.

DOSAGE: Oral Solution; Tablets; Tablets, Oral Disintegrating

Prevent N&V associated with moderately emetogenic cancer chemotherapy.

Children, over 12 years: One 8 mg tablet or orally disintegrating tablet or 10 mL (equivalent to 8 mg ondansetron) oral solution twice a day. Give the first dose 30 min before treatment followed by a second 8-mg dose 8 hr after the first dose; **then,** 8 mg twice a day for 1–2 days after chemotherapy. **4–11 years:** One 4 mg tablet or orally disintegrating tablet or 5 mL (equivalent to 4 mg ondansetron) oral solution 3 times per day. The first dose is given 30 min before chemotherapy with subsequent doses 4 and 8 hr after the first dose. **Then,** 4 mg q 8 hr for 1–2 days after completion of chemotherapy.

NEED TO KNOW

1. Safety and effectiveness in children 3 years and younger are not known.
2. There is no experience giving ondansetron to children to prevent postoperative N&V.
3. When IV is used to prevent chemotherapy-induced N&V, dilute the 2 mg/mL injection in 50 mL of D5W or 0.9% NaCl injection and infuse over 15 min.
4. Ondansetron injection, 2 mg/mL, requires no dilution for administration for postoperative N&V.
5. May be continued 1–2 days following chemotherapy to ensure prevention of N&V.
6. May cause drowsiness or dizziness.
7. Report any rash, diarrhea, constipation, altered respirations (bronchospasms), or loss of response.

Oseltamivir phosphate

(oh-sell-**TAM**-ih-vir)

Rx: Tamiflu.

C

CLASSIFICATION(S): Antiviral

USES: (1) Prophylaxis of influenza A and B in children, 1 year of age and older. (2) Treatment of uncomplicated acute influenza in children over 1 year of age who have been symptomatic for 2 days or less. *NOTE:* Oseltamivir is not a substitute for early vaccination on an annual basis as recommended by the CDC.

ACTION/KINETICS: May act by inhibiting the flu virus neuraminidase with possible alteration of virus particle aggregation and release. Readily absorbed from the GI tract and extensively converted to oseltamivir carboxylate. **$t_{1/2}$, oseltamivir:** 1–3 hr; **$t_{1/2}$, oseltamivir carboxylate:** 6–10 hr. Over 99% is eliminated in the urine as oseltamivir carboxylate. Children up to 12 years clear the prodrug and the active metabolite (carboxylate) faster than adults.

SIDE EFFECTS: Children: Diarrhea, N&V, abdominal pain, asthma, epistaxis, otitis media. *ANAPHYLAXIS* (rare).

DOSAGE: Capsules; Oral Suspension

Prophylaxis of influenza.

Children, 13 years and older: 75 mg once daily for at least 10 days. Begin treatment within 2 days of exposure to flu. **1 year and older following close contact with an infected individual: 15 kg or less (33 lbs or less):** 30 mg (2.4 mL of the suspension) twice a day; **15–23 kg (33–51 lbs):** 45 mg (3.6 mL of the suspension) twice a day; **23–40 kg (51–88 lbs):** 60 mg (4.8 mL of the suspension) twice a day; **greater than 40 kg (greater than 88 lbs):** 75 mg (6 mL of the suspension) twice a day. Prophylaxis in children has not been evaluated for longer than 10 days duration.

Treatment of influenza.

Children, 13 years and older: 75 mg twice a day for 5 days.

For clients with a C_{CR} between 10 and 30 mL/min, reduce dose to 75 mg once daily for 5 days. **1 year and older: 15 kg or less (33 lbs or less):** 30 mg (2.4 mL of the suspension) twice a day; **15–23 kg (33–51 lbs):** 45 mg (3.6 mL of the suspension) twice a day; **23–40 kg (51–88 lbs):** 60 mg (4.8 mL of the suspension) twice a day; **greater than 40 kg (greater than 88 lbs):** 75 mg (6 mL of the suspension) twice a day. Duration: 5 days.

NEED TO KNOW

1. Efficacy has not been determined in clients who begin treatment after 40 hr of symptoms, for prophylactic use to prevent influenza, for repeated treatment courses.
2. Safety and efficacy have not been determined in children less than 1 year of age or of repeated treatment or prophylaxis.
3. Use the reconstituted solution within 10 days of preparation.
4. Drug is used to diminish side effects and duration of illness. An annual flu shot is still required.
5. Do not double up on doses. Take any missed dose as soon as remembered. If the missed dose is remembered within 2 hr of the next scheduled dose, take at the usual time and resume usual schedule.
6. Tolerability may be enhanced if taken with food. May aggravate diabetes control.
7. May cause dizziness or lightheadedness; hot weather, exercise, or fever may increase effects.
8. An increased risk of confusion and unusual behavioral changes has been noted. The risk may be greater in children.

Oxcarbazepine

(ox-kar-**BAY**-zeh-peen)

Rx: Trileptal.

C

CLASSIFICATION(S): Anticonvulsant, miscellaneous

USES: (1) Monotherapy to treat partial seizures in children 4 years and older. (2) Adjunctive therapy to treat partial seizures in children 2 years and older.

ACTION/KINETICS: Effect is primarily through the active 10-monohydroxy metabolite. May block voltage-sensitive sodium channels, resulting in stabilization of hyperexcited neural membranes, inhibition of repetitive neuronal firing, and decreased propagation of synaptic impulses. These effects are thought to be important in preventing seizure spread. Completely absorbed and extensively metabolized to the active 10-monohydroxy metabolite (MHD). **Peak levels:** 4.5 hr for oxcarbazepine and 6 hr for MHD. Steady-state plasma levels reached in 2–3 days. **$t_{1/2}$, oxcarbazepine:** About 2 hr; **$t_{1/2}$, MHD:** About 9 hr. MHD and inactive metabolites are excreted mainly in the urine.

SIDE EFFECTS: Children: Headache, somnolence, dizziness, ataxia, nystagmus, N&V, rhinitis, diplopia, abnormal vision, fatigue.

DOSAGE:

Adjunctive therapy for partial seizure.

Children, 4–12 years, initial: 8–10 mg/kg, not to exceed 300 mg twice a day. Achieve target maintenance dose over 2 weeks according to client weight as follows: **20–29 kg:** 900 mg/day; **29.1–39 kg:** 1,200 mg/day; **over 39 kg:** 1,800 mg/day. **2–4 years, initial:** 8–10 mg/kg, not to exceed 300 mg twice a day. For those weighing less than 20 kg, consider a starting dose of 16–20 mg/kg. Achieve a target maintenance dose over 2 weeks, not to exceed 60 mg/kg/day as a twice daily regimen. *NOTE:* Children 2 to younger than 4 years may require twice the dose of oxcarbazpine per body weight compared with adults and children 4 to 12 years may require a 50% higher oxcarbazepine dose per body weight compared with adults.

Conversion to monotherapy.

Children, 4–16 years, initial: 8–10 mg/kg/day in 2 divided doses while simultaneously reducing the dose of the concomitant antiepileptic drug. The concomitant drug can be completely withdrawn over 3–6 weeks, while oxcarbazepine may be increased, up to a maximum increment of 10 mg/kg/day at approximately weekly intervals to reach the recommended daily dose.

Initiation of monotherapy.

Children, 4–16 years initial: 8–10 mg/kg/day in 2 divided doses. Increase the dose by 5 mg/kg/day every third day to the recommended daily maintenance dose as follows: **20 kg:** 600–900 mg/day; **25 kg and 30 kg:** 900–1,200 mg/day. **35 kg and 40 kg:** 900–1,500 mg/day; **45 kg:** 1,200–1,500 mg; **50 kg and 55 kg:** 1,200–1,800 mg/day; **60 kg and 65 kg:** 1,200–2,100 mg/day; **70 kg:** 1,500–2,100 mg/day.

NEED TO KNOW

1. If withdrawal is needed, do so gradually to prevent increased seizure frequency.
2. Take exactly as directed with or without food. Do not double or skip doses.
3. Shake oral suspension well. May mix with water or swallow directly from syringe.
4. May cause dizziness/drowsiness. Do not perform activities that require mental alertness until drug effects realized.

Palivizumab

(**pal**-ih-**VIZ**-you-mab)

Rx: Synagis.

C

CLASSIFICATION(S): Monoclonal antibody

USES: Prevention of serious lower respiratory tract disease due to RSV in pediatric clients at high risk of RSV disease. May be used (1) in children with hemodynamically significant congenital heart disease to prevent hospitalization due to RSV, (2) in infants with bronchopulmonary dysplasia, and (3) in infants 35 weeks or less gestational age.

ACTION/KINETICS: Exhibits neutralizing and fusion-inhibitory activity against respiratory syncytial virus (RSV), leading to a reduction in the quantity of RSV in the lower respiratory tract. **$t_{1/2}$, children:** 20 days.

SIDE EFFECTS: N&V, fever, URTI, otitis media, rhinitis, rash, pain, hernia, pharyngitis.

DOSAGE: IM

Prevention of RSV disease.

Children: 15 mg/kg per month IM (preferably in the anterolateral part of the thigh) throughout the RSV season. To calculate the monthly dose: client weight (kg) × 15 mg/kg divided by 100 mg/mL of palivizumab.

NEED TO KNOW

1. Safety and efficacy have not been determined for treatment of established RSV disease.
2. Give injection volumes greater than 1 mL in divided doses.
3. The injection does not have to be reconstituted and is available for injection immediately.
4. Reconstituted palivizumab does not contain a preservative; administer within 6 hr of reconstitution.
5. Give monthly doses throughout the RSV season. In the northern hemisphere, the RSV season usually begins in November and lasts through April.
6. Protect child from exposure to infection while on therapy (i.e., limit visitors, and avoid infected persons). Providers may need to wear masks and gloves.
7. May experience URI, runny nose, sore throat, ear infections, rash, or pain at injection site; report fever, other infections, and difficulty breathing.

Penicillin G Aqueous
(pen-ih-**SILL**-in)
Rx: Pfizerpen.

B

CLASSIFICATION(S): Antibiotic, penicillin
USES: Streptococci of groups A, C, G, H, L, and M are sensitive to penicillin G. High serum levels are effective against streptococci of the D group.
ACTION/KINETICS: Rapid onset makes it especially suitable for fulminating infections. Is neither penicillinase resistant nor acid stable. **Peak plasma levels: IM or SC,** 6–20 units/mL after 15–30 min. **t½:** 30 min.
SIDE EFFECTS: Hypersensitivity reactions, N&V, diarrhea, abdominal cramps, thrush/yeast infection, sore mouth/tongue.

DOSAGE: IM; IV, Infusion (Continuous)

Serious streptococcal infections (empyema, endocarditis, meningitis, pericarditis, pneumonia).

Children: 150,000 units/kg/day given in equal doses q 4 to 6 hr. **Infants over 7 days:** 75,000 units/kg/day in divided doses q 8 hr. **Infants less than 7 days:** 50,000 units/kg/day given in divided doses q 12 hr. For group B streptococcus, give 100,000 units/kg/day.

Meningitis due to susceptible strains of Pneumococcus *or* Meningococcus.

Children: 250,000 units/kg/day divided in equal doses q 4 to 6 hr for 7 to 14 days (maximum total daily dose: 12–20 million units). **Infants over 7 days:** 200,000–300,0000 units/kg/day divided into equal doses given q 6 hr. **Infants less than 7 days:** 100,000–150,000 units/kg/day.

Rat-bite fever, Haverhill fever.

Children: 150,000–250,000 units/kg/day in equal doses q 4 hr for 4 weeks.

Adjunct with antitoxin to prevent diphtheria.

Children: 150,000–250,000 units/kg/day in equal doses q 6 hr for 7–10 days.

Disseminated gonococcal infections.

Children, less than 45 kg: *Arthritis:* 100,000 units/kg/day in 4 equally divided doses for 7 to 10 days. *Endocarditis:* 250,000 units/kg/day in equal doses q 4 hr for 4 weeks. *Meningitis:* 250,000 units/kg/day in equal doses q 4 hr for 10 to 14 days. **Over 45 kg:** *Arthritis, endocarditis, meningitis:* 10 million units/day in 4 equally divided doses (duration depends on type of infection).

Symptomatic or asymptomatic congenital syphilis in infants.

Infants: 50,000 units/kg/dose IV q 12 hr the first 7 days; then, q 8 hr for a total of 10 days. **Children:** 50,000 units/kg q 4–6 hr for 10 days.

NEED TO KNOW

1. IM administration is preferred; discomfort is minimized by using solutions of up to 100,000 units/mL. Keep the total volume of the IM injection small.
2. The preferred route in bacterial meningitis is IV supplemented by IM.
3. Assess drug allergies.
4. Monitor I&O. Dehydration decreases drug excretion and may raise blood level of penicillin G to dangerously high levels, causing kidney damage. GI disturbances may lead to dehydration.
5. With IM dosing may experience pain at injection site; apply ice to relieve pain.
6. Report any unusual bruising, bleeding, N&V, sore mouth, diarrhea, rash, fever, difficulty breathing, adverse side effects, or lack of improvement.

Penicillin G benzathine, intramuscular ■ B

(pen-ih-**SILL**-in, **BEN**-zah-theen)

Rx: Bicillin L-A, Permapen.

CLASSIFICATION(S): Antibiotic, penicillin
USES: (1) URTI (mild to moderate) due to susceptible streptococci. (2) Sexually transmitted diseases, such as syphilis, yaws, bejel, and pinta. (3) Follow-up prophylactic therapy for rheumatic heart disease and acute glomerulonephritis.
ACTION/KINETICS: Penicillin G is neither penicillinase resistant nor acid stable. **Peak plasma levels, IM:** 0.03–0.05 unit/mL.
SIDE EFFECTS: Hypersensitivity reactions, N&V, diarrhea, abdominal cramps, thrush/yeast infection, sore mouth/tongue.

DOSAGE: IM Only (Suspension)

URTI due to Group A streptococcus.
Older children: 900,000 units as a single dose; **children, under 27 kg:** 300,000–600,000 units as a single dose.

Early syphilis (primary, secondary, or latent).
Children: 50,000 units/kg, up to a single dose of 2,4000,000 units.

Gummas and cardiovascular syphilis (latent).
Children: 50,000 units/kg, up to 2,400,000 units q 7 days for 3 weeks.

Congenital syphilis.
Children, 2–12 years: Adjust dose based on adult dosage schedule.

Prophylaxis of rheumatic fever and glomerulonephritis.
Following an acute attack, 1,200,000 units once a month or 600,000 units q 2 weeks.

NEED TO KNOW

1. This product is not intended for IV administration.
2. Inject slowly and steadily into muscle; *do not massage* injection site. For infants and small children, the midlateral aspect

of the thigh should be used. Do not administer in the gluteal region in children less than 2 years. Rotate and chart site of injections. Divide between two injection sites if dose is large or available muscle mass is small.

3. Report any unusual side effects, lack of response or worsening of condition.

Penicillin V potassium

(pen-ih-**SILL**-in)

Rx: Penicillin VK, Veetids.

B

CLASSIFICATION(S): Antibiotic, penicillin

USES: (1) Mild to moderate upper respiratory tract streptococcal infections, including scarlet fever and erysipelas. (2) Mild to moderate upper respiratory tract pneumococcal infections, including otitis media. (3) Mild staphylococcal infections of the skin and soft tissue. (4) Mild to moderate fusospirochetosis (Vincent's infection) of the oropharynx, pharyngitis. (5) Prophylaxis of recurrence following rheumatic fever or chorea.

ACTION/KINETICS: Binds to penicillin-binding proteins (PBP-1 and PBP-3) in the cytoplasmic membranes of bacteria, thus inhibiting cell wall synthesis. Cell division and growth are inhibited and often lysis and elongation of susceptible bacteria occur. Products are not penicillinase resistant but are acid stable and resist inactivation by gastric secretions. Well absorbed from the GI tract and not affected by foods. **Peak plasma levels: PO:** 1–9 mcg/mL after 30–60 min. **t½:** 30 min.

SIDE EFFECTS: Hypersensitivity reactions, N&V, diarrhea, abdominal cramps, thrush/yeast infection, sore mouth/tongue.

DOSAGE: Oral Solution; Tablets

Streptococcal infections of the upper respiratory tract, including scarlet fever and mild erysipelas.

Children, over 12 years: 125–250 mg q 6–8 hr for 10 days.

Pharyngitis in children, usual: 25–50 mg/kg/day divided q 6 hr for 10 days.

Staphylococcal infections (mild infections of the skin and soft tissue); fusospirochetosis of oropharynx (mild to moderate infections).

Children, over 12 years: 250 mg q 6–8 hr.

Pneumococcal infections, mild to moderate respiratory tract infections, including otitis media.

Children, over 12 years: 250 mg q 6 hr until afebrile for at least 2 days.

Prophylaxis of recurrence of rheumatic fever/chorea.

Children, over 12 years: 125–250 mg twice a day, on a continuing basis.

Prophylactic treatment of children with sickle cell anemia or splenectomy to reduce incidence of S. pneumoniae *septicemia.*

Children, 3 months–5 years: 125 mg twice a day. **Over 5 years:** 250 mg twice a day.

Anthrax, postexposure prophylaxis (confirmed or suspected exposure to B. anthracis*).*

Children, less than 9 years: 50 mg/kg/day divided 4 times per day. Continue prophylaxis until exposure to *B. anthracis* has been excluded. If exposure is confirmed and vaccine is available, continue prophylaxis for 4 weeks and until 3 doses of vaccine have been given or for 30–60 days if vaccine is not available.

Early Lyme disease (Borrelia burgdorferi).

Children, over 12 years: 500 mg 4 times per day for 10–20 days.

NEED TO KNOW

1. More and more strains of staphylococci are resistant to penicillin V, necessitating culture and sensitivity studies.
2. Store reconstituted solution in the refrigerator; discard unused portion after 14 days.
3. Take without regard to meals. Blood levels may be slightly

higher when administered on an empty stomach. Take after meals to enhance absorption.

4. Report lack of response, adverse side effects, bloody stools, severe diarrhea, or stomach cramps/pain or if throat/ear symptoms do not improve after 48 hr of therapy; may need to reevaluate and alter therapy.
5. With oral administration, if reaction is going to occur, it usually occurs after the second dose. Seek medical intervention immediately if respiratory distress or skin wheals appear.

Phenobarbital

(fee-no-**BAR**-bih-tal)

Rx: Bellatal, Solfoton, **C-IV.**

Phenobarbital sodium

Rx: Luminal Sodium, **C-IV.**

D

CLASSIFICATION(S): Sedative-hypnotic, barbiturate

USES: PO: (1) Sedative or hypnotic (short-term). (2) Anticonvulsant (partial and generalized tonic-clonic or cortical focal seizures). (3) Emergency control of acute seizure disorders due to status epilepticus, meningitis, tetanus, eclampsia, toxicity of local anesthetics. **Parenteral:** (1) Preanesthetic. (2) Anticonvulsant (generalized tonic-clonic and cortical focal seizures). (3) Emergency control of acute seizure disorders (e.g., tetanus, eclampsia, status epilepticus).

ACTION/KINETICS: Depressant and anticonvulsant effects may be related to its ability to increase and/or mimic the inhibitory activity of GABA on nerve synapses. **Onset:** 30 to more than 60 min. **Duration:** 10–16 hr. **Anticonvulsant therapeutic serum levels:** 15–40 mcg/mL. **Time for peak effect, after IV:** Up to 15 min. Distributed more slowly than other barbiturates due to lower lipid solubility. Long-acting. **t½:** 53–140 hr. Twenty-five percent eliminated unchanged in the urine. **Plasma protein binding:** 50–60%.

SIDE EFFECTS: Somnolence, headache, agitation, confusion, ataxia, dizziness, pain at injection site. *APNEA, RESPIRATORY DEPRESSION, ANGIODEMA.*

DOSAGE: Capsules; Elixir; Tablets PHENOBARBITAL, PHENOBARBITAL SODIUM

Sedation.

Children: 8–32 mg.

Hypnotic.

Children: Dose should be determined by provider, based on age and weight.

Anticonvulsant.

Children: 3–6 mg/kg/day in single or divided doses. In infants and children, a loading dose of 15–20 mg/kg achieves blood levels of about 20 mcg/mL shortly after administration. To reach therapeutic blood levels of 10–25 mcg/mL, higher doses per kilogram are generally necessary compared with adults.

DOSAGE: IM; IV

Preoperative sedation.

Children: 1–3 mg/kg IM or IV 60–90 min prior to surgery.

Acute convulsions.

Children: 4–6 mg/kg/day for 7–10 days to achieve a blood level of 10–15 mcg/mL (or 10–15 mg/kg/day, IV or IM).

Status epilepticus.

Children: 15–20 mg/kg given over a 10 to 15 min period. *NOTE:* Use the minimal amount required and wait for the anticonvulsant effect to occur before giving a second dose.

NEED TO KNOW

1. When given in the presence of pain, restlessness, excitement, and delirium may result.
2. Use parenterally only when PO use is impossible or impractical.
3. When used for seizures, give major part of the dose according

to when seizures are likely to occur (i.e., on arising for daytime seizures; at bedtime when seizures occur at night).

4. In most cases, when used for epilepsy, drug must be taken regularly to avoid seizures, even when no seizures are imminent. Give lowest dose possible to avoid adding to the depression that may follow seizures.
5. May initially cause drowsiness; assess effects before performing tasks that require mental alertness.
6. Do not stop abruptly following long-term use; may precipitate seizures. Tolerance may develop and require dosage adjustment.
7. Report any loss of effects, adverse effects or fever, sore throat, rash or bruising/bleeding. Brush teeth frequently and carefully to prevent gingivitis.

Phenytoin **C**
(**FEN**-ih-toyn)
Rx: Dilantin Infatab, Dilantin-125.
Phenytoin sodium, extended
Rx: Dilantin Kapseals, Phenytek.
Phenytoin sodium, parenteral
Rx: Dilantin Sodium.
Phenytoin sodium prompt
Rx: Diphenylan Sodium.

CLASSIFICATION(S): Anticonvulsant, hydantoin
USES: (1) Chronic epilepsy, especially of the tonic-clonic, psychomotor type. Not effective against absence seizures and may even increase the frequency of seizures in this disorder. (2) **Parenteral:** Status epilepticus and to control seizures during neurosurgery.
ACTION/KINETICS: Acts in the motor cortex of the brain to reduce the spread of electrical discharges from the rapidly firing epi-

leptic foci in this area. This is accomplished by stabilizing hyperexcitable cells possibly by affecting sodium efflux. Also, phenytoin decreases activity of centers in the brain stem responsible for the tonic phase of grand mal seizures. Has few sedative effects. It has a slow dissolution rate. Absorption is variable following PO dosage. **Peak serum levels, PO:** 4–8 hr. Since the rate and extent of absorption depend on the particular preparation, the same product should be used for a particular client. **Peak serum levels, IM:** 24 hr (wide variation). **Therapeutic serum levels:** 5–20 mcg/mL. **t½:** 8–60 hr (average: 20–30 hr). **Steady state:** 7–10 days after initiation. Both inactive metabolites and unchanged (less than 5%) drug are excreted in the urine.

SIDE EFFECTS: Ataxia, drowsiness, slurred speech, confusion, N&V, rash, constipation/diarrhea, gingival hyperplasia, *INCREASED SEIZURES, AGRANULOCYTOSIS, APLASTIC ANEMIA, HEMOLYTIC ANEMIA, RAPID PARENTERAL ADMINISTRATION MAY CAUSE SERIOUS CV EFFECTS.*

DOSAGE: Oral Suspension; Tablets, Chewable

Seizures.

Children, initial: 5 mg/kg/day in two to three divided doses; **maintenance,** 4–8 mg/kg (up to maximum of 300 mg/day). Children over 6 years may require up to 300 mg/day.

DOSAGE: Capsules; Capsules, Extended-Release

Children: See dose for Oral Suspension and Chewable Tablets.

DOSAGE: IV

Status epilepticus.

Children, loading dose: 15–20 mg/kg in divided doses of 5–10 mg/kg given at a rate of 1–3 mg/kg/min.

DOSAGE: IM

Neurosurgery.

Dose should be 50% greater than the PO dose.

NEED TO KNOW

1. Administer with extreme caution to clients with a history of asthma or other allergies, impaired renal or hepatic function.
2. Abrupt withdrawal may cause status epilepticus.

3. Full effectiveness of PO administered hydantoins is delayed and may take 6–9 days to be fully established. A similar period of time will elapse before effects disappear completely.
4. Avoid IM, SC, or perivascular injections.
5. Due to potential differences in bioavailability between PO products, do not interchange brands. Also, when switching from extended to prompt products, dosage adjustments may be required.
6. Use of IV infusion is not recommended, as the drug is poorly soluble and may form a precipitate.
7. *Do not* add phenytoin to an already running IV solution.
8. If IV is used, a rate of 1–3 mg/kg/min should not be exceeded in neonates.
9. May take with food to minimize GI upset. Do not take antacids within 1 hr of ingestion. Do not chew or crush; take tablets whole.
10. If dose is missed, take as soon as remembered. Then resume the usual schedule. Do not double up to make up for the missed dose.
11. To minimize bleeding from the gums and prevent gingival hyperplasia, practice good oral hygiene. Brush teeth with a soft toothbrush, massage the gums, and floss every day. Advise dentist of therapy.
12. Responsible for a large number of potential drug interactions; monitor carefully if given with other drugs.

Pravastatin sodium

(prah-vah-**STAH**-tin)

Rx: Pravachol. **X**

CLASSIFICATION(S): Antihyperlipidemic, HMG-CoA reductase inhibitor

USES: Adjunct to diet and lifestyle modification to treat heterozygous familial hypercholesterolemia in children 8 years and older if after an adequate trial of diet the following are present: LDL-C remains 190 mg/dL or greater or LDL-C remains 160 mg/dL and there is a positive family history of premature CV disease or 2 or more other cardiovascular disease factors are present.

ACTION/KINETICS: Competitively inhibits HMG-CoA reductase; this enzyme catalyzes the early rate-limiting step in the synthesis of cholesterol. Thus, cholesterol synthesis is inhibited/decreased. Decreases total cholesterol, triglycerides, LDL, and VLDL and increases HDL. Rapidly absorbed from the GI tract. **Peak plasma levels:** 1–1.5 hr. Significant first-pass extraction and metabolism in the liver, which is the site of action of the drug; thus, plasma levels may not correlate well with lipid-lowering effectiveness. **t½, elimination:** 77 hr. Metabolized in the liver; excreted in the urine (about 20%) and feces (70%).

SIDE EFFECTS: Localized pain, N&V, diarrhea, abdominal cramps/pain, constipation, flatulence, fatigue, flu syndrome, common cold, rhinitis, rash/pruritus, cardiac chest pain, dizziness, headache.

DOSAGE: Tablets

Antihyperlipidemic.

Children, 8–13 years (inclusive): 20 mg once daily. Doses greater than 20 mg have not been studied in this population. **14–18 years, initial:** 40 mg once daily. Doses greater than 40 mg have not been studied in this population.

NEED TO KNOW

1. Place on a standard cholesterol-lowering diet for 3–6 months before beginning pravastatin and continue during therapy, unless more than 3 risk factors.
2. Drug may be taken without regard to meals.
3. The maximum effect is seen within 4 weeks during which time periodic lipid determinations should be undertaken.
4. Pravastatin should be discontinued if markedly elevated CPK levels occur or myopathy is diagnosed.
5. Take as directed at bedtime.

6. Report severe GI upset, unusual bruising/bleeding, vision changes, dark urine, or light colored stools.
7. Avoid prolonged or excessive exposure to direct or artificial sunlight.

Prednisolone **C**
(pred-**NISS**-oh-lohn)
Rx: Syrup: Prelone. **Tablets:** Delta-Cortef.
Prednisolone sodium phosphate
Rx: Oral Liquid/Solution: Pediapred. **Oral Solution:** Orapred. **Tablets, Orally Disintegrating:** Orapred ODT.
Prednisolone tebutate
Rx: Prednisol TPA.

CLASSIFICATION(S): Glucocorticoid
ACTION/KINETICS: Is five times more potent than hydrocortisone and cortisone. Minimal side effects except for GI distress. Moderate mineralocorticoid activity. **Plasma $t^1/_2$:** over 200 min.
SIDE EFFECTS: Insomnia, N&V, GI upset, fatigue, dizziness, muscle weakness, increased hunger/thirst, joint pain, decreased diabetic control.

DOSAGE: Syrup; Tablets PREDNISOLONE
Most uses.
5–60 mg/day, depending on disease being treated.
DOSAGE: Injection, Soft Tissue; Intra-articular; Intralesional
4–100 mg (larger doses for large joints).
DOSAGE: Oral Liquid/Solution PREDNISOLONE SODIUM PHOSPHATE
Most uses.
5–60 mg/day in single or divided doses.

Adrenocortical insufficiency.

Children: 0.14 mg/kg (4 mg/m^2) daily in three to four divided doses.

Other pediatric uses.

0.5–2 mg/kg (15–60 mg/m^2) daily in three to four divided doses.

DOSAGE: Tablets, Orally Disintegrating

10–60 mg/day (prednisolone base).

DOSAGE: Injection, Soft Tissue; Intra-articular; Intralesional

PREDNISOLONE TEBUTATE

4–30 mg, depending on site and severity of disease. Doses higher than 40 mg are not recommended.

NEED TO KNOW

1. Use with particular caution in diabetes.
2. Before administering, check spelling and dose carefully; frequently confused with prednisone.
3. Shake suspension well before using.
4. Take as directed and do not stop suddenly without provider approval; adrenal crisis may occur.
5. May take with food to decrease GI upset. Report any loss of effect; dose may need adjustment.
6. Report nausea, anorexia, fatigue, joint pain, weakness, dizziness, or SOB; S&S of adrenal insufficiency.
7. Assess for weight gain, swelling of extremities, and adjust diet/salt intake and exercise to control.

Prednisone **C**

(**PRED**-nih-sohn)

Rx: Oral Solution: Prednisone Intensol Concentrate. **Syrup**: Liquid Pred. **Tablets**: Deltasone, Meticorten, Orasone, Panasol-S, Prednicen-M, Sterapred, Sterapred DS.

CLASSIFICATION(S): Glucocorticoid

USES: (1) Adrenal insufficiency. (2) Congenital adrenal hyperplasia.

(3) Asthma. (4) Allergic reactions. (5) Acute leukemia. (6) Nephrotic syndrome.

ACTION/KINETICS: The anti-inflammatory effect is due to inhibition of prostaglandin synthesis. The drug also inhibits accumulation of macrophages and leukocytes at sites of inflammation and inhibits phagocytosis and lysosomal enzyme release. Three to five times as potent as cortisone or hydrocortisone. May cause moderate fluid retention. Metabolized in the liver to prednisolone, the active form.

SIDE EFFECTS: Insomnia, N&V, GI upset, fatigue, dizziness, muscle weakness, increased hunger/thirst, joint pain, decreased diabetic control.

DOSAGE: Oral Solution; Syrup; Tablets

Acute, severe conditions.

Initial: 5–60 mg/day in four equally divided doses after meals and at bedtime. Decrease gradually by 5–10 mg q 4–5 days to establish minimum maintenance dosage (5–10 mg) or discontinue altogether until symptoms recur.

Replacement.

Children: 0.1–0.15 mg/kg/day.

NEED TO KNOW

1. Take in the morning to prevent insomnia and with food to decrease GI upset.
2. Do not stop abruptly with long-term therapy. Take as directed and wean as directed.
3. Report any S&S of adrenal insufficiency (N&V, confusion, appetite loss, low BP), loss of effectiveness.
4. With long-term therapy may experience cataracts, glaucoma, eye infections, bone weakening which may lead to osteoporosis, elevation in BP, diabetes, salt and water retention, and increased potassium loss. Consume adequate calcium and vitamin D supplements.

Primaquine phosphate (PRIM-ah-kwin)

C

CLASSIFICATION(S): Antimalarial, 8-aminoquinolone

USES: (1) Radical cure of *Plasmodium vivax* malaria. (2) Prophylaxis of relapse in *P. vivax* malaria.

ACTION/KINETICS: Mechanism of action not known, but the drug binds to and may alter the properties of DNA leading to decreased protein synthesis. Both the gametocyte and exoerythrocyte forms are inhibited. Well absorbed from GI tract. **Peak plasma levels:** 1–3 hr. Poorly distributed in body tissues. **t½, elimination:** 4 hr. Rapidly metabolized.

SIDE EFFECTS: N&V, abdominal cramps, epigastric distress, leukopenia.

DOSAGE: Tablets

Acute attack of vivax malaria, clients with parasitized RBCs.

26.3 mg (15 mg base) daily for 14 days together with chloroquine phosphate (to destroy erythrocytic parasites).

Suppression of malaria.

Children: 0.5 mg/kg/day (0.3 mg/kg base) for 14 days.

NEED TO KNOW

1. Do not use with other bone marrow depressants or hemolytic drugs.
2. For suppression therapy, initiate during the last 2 weeks of or after suppressive therapy with chloroquine or a similar drug.
3. Obtain hematologic profile and cultures. Monitor for indications to withdraw drug: dark urine may indicate hemolysis.
4. Assess dark-skinned clients closely. Because of a possible inborn deficiency of G6PD, these clients are particularly susceptible to hemolytic anemia while on primaquine.
5. Take immediately before or after meals or with antacids to minimize gastric irritation.
6. Report any GI, neurologic, and cardiovascular disturbances; symptoms of overdose.

Promethazine hydrochloride ■ C
(proh-**METH**-ah-zeen)
Rx: Phenadoz, Phenergen.

CLASSIFICATION(S): Antihistamine, first generation, phenothiazine
USES: PO, Rectal. (1) Perennial and seasonal allergic rhinitis; vasomotor rhinitis. (2) Allergic conjunctivitis due to inhalant allergens and foods. (3) Mild, uncomplicated allergic skin manifestations of urticaria and angioedema. (4) Relief of allergic reactions to blood or plasma. (5) Adjunct to epinephrine and other measures to treat anaphylactic reactions after acute symptoms have been controlled. (6) Preoperative, postoperative sedation. (7) Prevention and control of N&V associated with certain types of anesthesia and surgery. (8) Sedation in children. (9) Active and prophylactic treatment of motion sickness. (10) Antiemetic in postoperative clients. **Parenteral.** (1) Adjunct to control postoperative pain. (2) Prevention and control of N&V associated with certain types of anesthesia and surgery and in postoperative clients. (3) Type I hypersensitivity reactions, including perennial and seasonal allergic rhinitis; vasomotor rhinitis; allergic conjunctivitis due to inhalant allergens and foods; mild, uncomplicated allergic skin reactions of urticaria and angioedema; amelioration of allergic reactions due to blood or plasma; dermatographism; adjunctive anaphylactic therapy. (4) Preoperative, postoperative sedation. (5) Use parenteral therapy when PO therapy is impossible or contraindicated.
ACTION/KINETICS: Antiemetic effects are likely due to inhibition of the CTZ. Effective in vertigo by its central anticholinergic effect which inhibits the vestibular apparatus and the integrative vomiting center as well as the CTZ. May cause severe drowsiness. **Onset, PO, IM, PR:** 20 min; **IV:** 3–5 min. **Duration, antihistaminic:** 6–12 hr; **sedative:** 2–8 hr. Slowly eliminated through urine and feces.
SIDE EFFECTS: Drowsiness, dizziness, confusion, blurred vision,

dry mouth, tinnitus, N&V, photosensitivity. *RESPIRATORY DEPRESSION, APNEA.*

DOSAGE: Suppositories; Syrup; Tablets

Allergies.

Children, over 2 years: 25 mg at bedtime (usual dose); 12.5 mg before meals and at bedtime may be given, if needed. Single 25 mg doses at bedtime or 6.25–12.5 mg taken 3 times per day will usually suffice. Adjust dose to the smallest amount needed to relieve symptoms. If given rectally, resume PO administration as soon as possible if continued therapy is needed.

Sedation.

Children, over 2 years: 12.5–25 mg at bedtime. *NOTE:* If used for preoperative sedation, give the night before surgery to relieve apprehension and to produce quiet sleep.

Antiemetic.

Children, over 2 years: 25 mg or 0.5 mg/lb (usual dose); doses of 12.5–25 mg may be repeated q 4–6 hr as needed for prophylaxis and treatment of active N&V. Adjust dose to the age, weight, and severity of the condition of the client. Limit use to prolonged vomiting of known etiology.

Motion sickness.

Children, over 2 years: 12.5–25 mg twice a day.

Pre- and postoperative use.

Children, over 2 years: 0.5 mg/lb (1.2 mg/kg) preoperatively in combination with an appropriately reduced dose of narcotic or barbiturate and the appropriate dose of an atropine-like drug. Give 12.5–25 mg for postoperative sedation and adjunctive use with analgesics. To produce quiet sleep and to relieve apprehension, give 12.5–25 mg the night before surgery.

DOSAGE: IM (Preferred); IV

Hypersensitivity reactions, Type I.

Children, 2 years and older: Do not exceed one-half the adult dose (25 mg; may repeat dose within 2 hr).

Sedation.

Children, 2–12 years: Do not exceed one-half the adult dose (25–50 mg at bedtime for nighttime sedation).

Antiemetic.

Children, 2–12 years: Do not exceed one-half the adult dose (12.5–25 mg). Do not use when etiology of vomiting is unknown.

Pre- and postoperative use.

Children, 2–12 years: 0.5 mg/lb (1.2 mg/kg) in combination with appropriately reduced doses of narcotic or barbiturate and atropine-like drugs.

NEED TO KNOW

1. Do not use promethazine in children younger than 2 years because of the potential for fatal respiratory depression.
2. Exercise caution when administering promethazine to children 2 years and older. It is recommended that the lowest effective dose of promethazine be used in children 2 years and older and that concomitant administration of other drugs with respiratory depressant effects should be avoided.
3. Do not use in children whose signs and symptoms may suggest Reye's syndrome or other hepatic diseases.
4. Use in children may cause paradoxical hyperexcitability and nightmares.
5. When used as adjunct to analgesics be aware it has no analgesic ability (only sedative effects) which may be pronounced.
6. Take only as directed and do not exceed dose; cardiac arrhythmias may occur. May take with food or milk to decrease GI upset.
7. Drug may alter skin testing; stop 72 hr before testing.
8. Consume adequate fluids to prevent dehydration; use caution in hot weather to prevent heat stroke.
9. Avoid prolonged sun exposure; may cause photosensitivity reaction. Wear sunscreen and protection if exposed.

Pseudoephedrine hydrochloride **B**
(soo-doh-eh-**FED**-rin)

OTC: Capsules: Sinustop. **Capsules, Soft Gel:** Dimetapp Maximum Strength Non-Drowsy Liqui-Gels. **Drops:** Dimetapp Decongestant Pediatric, Kid Kare, Nasal Decongestant Oral, PediaCare Decongestant Infants'. **Liquid/Syrup:** Cenafed Syrup, Decofed Syrup, ElixSure Children's Congestion, Simply Stuffy, Sudafed Children's Non-Drowsy, Triaminic Allergy Congestion, Unifed. **Tablets:** Cenafed, Congestaid, Genaphed, Medi-First Sinus Decongestant, Simply Stuffy, Sudafed Non-Drowsy Maximum Strength, Sudodrin. **Tablets, Chewable:** Sudafed Children's Non-Drowsy, Triaminic Allergy Congestion Softchews. **Tablets, Controlled Release or Extended-Release:** Dimetapp Maximum Strength 12-Hour Non-Drowsy Extentabs, Efidac 24 Pseudoephedrine, Sudafed Non-Drowsy 12 Hour Long-Acting, Sudafed Non-Drowsy 24 Hour Long-Acting.

Pseudoephedrine sulfate

OTC: Drixoral 12 Hour Non-Drowsy Formula.

CLASSIFICATION(S): Sympathomimetic

USES: Temporary relief of nasal congestion due to hay fever, common cold, or other upper respiratory allergies associated with sinusitis.

ACTION/KINETICS: Produces direct stimulation of both alpha- (pronounced) and beta-adrenergic receptors, as well as indirect stimulation through release of norepinephrine from storage sites. Results in decongestant effect on the nasal mucosa. **Onset:** 15–30 min. **Time to peak effect:** 30–60 min. **Duration:** 3–4 hr. **Extended-release, duration:** 8–12 hr. Urinary excretion slowed by alkalinization, causing reabsorption of drug.

SIDE EFFECTS: Somnolence, insomnia, nervousness, excitability, dizziness, anxiety, skin rashes, nausea, gastric irritation.

DOSAGE: Capsules; Capsules, Soft Gel; Drops; Liquid/Syrup; Tablets; Tablets, Chewable PSEUDOEPHEDRINE HYDROCHLORIDE

Decongestant.

Children, over 12 years: 60 mg q 4–6 hr, not to exceed 240 mg in 24 hr. **6–12 years:** 30 mg using the drops, liquid, syrup or chewable tablets q 4–6 hr, not to exceed 120 mg in 24 hr. **2–6 years:** Use not recommended.

DOSAGE: Tablets, Controlled-Release (24 hr); Tablets, Extended-Release (12 hr)

Decongestant.

Children, over 12 years: 120 mg of the sustained-release q 12 hr or 240 mg of the controlled-release q 24 hr. Do not exceed 240 mg/24 hr.

DOSAGE: Tablets, Extended-Release PSEUDOEPHEDRINE SULFATE

Decongestant.

Children, over 12 years: 120 mg q 12 hr, not to exceed 240 mg/24 hr. Use is not recommended for children less than 12 years.

NEED TO KNOW

1. Not recommended for use in children less than 6 years. Do not use sustained-release products in children less than 12 years.
2. Avoid taking near bedtime; stimulation may produce insomnia.
3. Take exactly as directed. Do not crush or chew extended-release products. Continuous use or excessive dosing may cause rebound congestion.
4. Report if symptoms do not improve after 3–5 days or worsen. Identify triggers and practice avoidance especially with seasonal allergies.

Pyrantel pamoate

(pie-**RAN**-tell)

OTC: Pin-Rid, Pin-X, Reese's Pinworm.

C

CLASSIFICATION(S): Anthelmintic

USES: (1) Pinworm (enterobiasis) and roundworm (ascariasis) infestations. (2) Multiple helminth infections, as it is also effective against roundworm and hookworm.

ACTION/KINETICS: Has neuromuscular blocking effect which paralyzes the helminth, allowing it to be expelled through the feces. Also inhibits cholinesterases. Poorly absorbed from GI tract. **Peak plasma levels:** 0.05–0.13 mcg/mL after 1–3 hr. Partially metabolized in liver.

SIDE EFFECTS: Anorexia, N&V, diarrhea, headache, dizziness.

DOSAGE: Capsules, Soft Gel; Liquid; Oral Suspension; Tablets

Pinworm, other helminth infections.

Children: One dose of 11 mg/kg (maximum). **Maximum total dose:** 1.0 gram.

NEED TO KNOW

1. Safe use in children less than 2 years has not been established.
2. May be taken without regard to food intake. Can take with milk or fruit juices.
3. Dizziness or drowsiness may occur; do not engage in activities that require mental alertness.
4. Purging is not required. Report rash, severe headaches/GI upset, joint pain, or prolonged dizziness.

Ranitidine hydrochloride
(rah-**NIH**-tih-deen)

B

OTC: Zantac 150 Maximum Strength Acid Reducer, Zantac 75 Acid Reducer. **Rx:** Zantac, Zantac EFFERdose.

CLASSIFICATION(S): Histamine H_2 receptor blocking drug
USES: Rx: (1) Short-term (4–8 weeks) and maintenance treatment of duodenal ulcer. (2) Pathologic hypersecretory conditions such as Zollinger-Ellison syndrome and systemic mastocytosis. (3) Short-term treatment of active, benign gastric ulcers and maintenance treatment after healing of the acute ulcer. (4) Treatment of GERD. (5) Treatment of endoscopically diagnosed erosive esophagitis and for maintenance of healing of erosive esophagitis. **OTC:** (1) Relief of heartburn associated with acid indigestion and sour stomach. (2) Prophylaxis of heartburn associated with acid indigestion and sour stomach due to certain foods and beverages.
ACTION/KINETICS: Competitively inhibits gastric acid secretion by blocking the effect of histamine on histamine H_2 receptors. Both daytime and nocturnal basal gastric acid secretion, as well as food- and pentagastrin-stimulated gastric acid are inhibited. Food increases the bioavailability. **Peak effect, PO:** 2–3 hr; **IM; IV:** 15 min. **t½:** 2.5–3 hr. **Duration, nocturnal:** 13 hr; **basal:** 4 hr. **Serum level to inhibit 50% stimulated gastric acid secretion:** 36–94 ng/mL. From 30% to 35% of a PO dose and from 68% to 79% of an IV dose excreted unchanged in urine.
SIDE EFFECTS: Headache, abdominal pain, constipation, diarrhea, N&V. *AGRANULOCYTOSIS, APLASTIC ANEMIA, BRONCHOSPASM, ANAPHYLAXIS.*

DOSAGE: Rx: Capsules; Syrup; Tablets; Tablets, Effervescent

Duodenal ulcer, short-term.

Children: 2–4 mg/kg/day given twice a day, up to a maximum of 300 mg/day. For maintenance in children, 2–4 mg/kg once daily, up to a maximum of 150 mg/day.

Pathologic hypersecretory conditions.

Children: 5–10 mg/kg/day, usually in 2 divided doses.

Benign gastric ulcer.

Children: 2–4 mg/kg/day given twice a day, up to a maximum of 300 mg/day. For maintenance in children, 2–4 mg/kg once daily, up to a maximum of 150 mg/day.

Gastroesophageal reflux disease.

Children: 5–10 mg/kg/day, usually given as 2 divided doses.

Maintenance of healing of erosive esophagitis.

Children: 5–10 mg/kg/day, usually in 2 divided doses.

DOSAGE: IM; IV

Treatment and maintenance for duodenal ulcer, hypersecretory conditions, gastroesophageal reflux.

Children, IV: 2–4 mg/kg/day in divided doses q 6–8 hr, up to a maximum of 50 mg q 6–8 hr.

DOSAGE: OTC: Tablets

Treat heartburn.

Treatment: 75 mg or 150 mg with a glass of water. **Maintenance:** Use up to 2 times per day (up to 2 tablets in 24 hr).

NEED TO KNOW

1. Give antacids concomitantly for gastric pain although they may interfere with ranitidine absorption.
2. Dissolve EFFERdose tablets and granules in 6–8 oz of water before taking. The 25 mg EFFERdose tablets (for use in infants) are dissolved in at least 5 mL of water; solution may be given with dosing cup, medicine dropper, or oral syringe.
3. About one-half of clients may heal completely within 2 weeks; thus, endoscopy may show no need for further treatment.
4. The premixed injection does not require dilution; give by slow IV drip over 15–20 min. Do not introduce additives into the solution.
5. Take as directed with or immediately following meals. Wait 1 hr before taking an antacid.
6. Report any evidence of yellow discoloration of skin or eyes, or diarrhea. Maintain adequate hydration. Report any confusion/

disorientation, unusual bruising or bleeding, black tarry stools, diarrhea, or rash immediately.

Respiratory Syncytial Virus Immune Globulin Intravenous (RSV-IGIV) (Human) C

Rx: RespiGam.

CLASSIFICATION(S): Immunosuppressant

USES: Prevention of serious lower respiratory tract infection caused by RSV in children, less than 24 months old with broncho-pulmonary dysplasia or a history of premature birth (less than 35 weeks gestation).

ACTION/KINETICS: An IgG containing neutralizing antibody to RSV. The immunoglobulin is obtained and purified from pooled adult human plasma that has been selected for high titers of neutralizing antibody against RSV.

SIDE EFFECTS: Fever, respiratory distress, vomiting, wheezing, diarrhea, rales, fluid overload, tachycardia, rash, hypertension, hypoxia, tachypnea, gastroenteritis, injection site reaction. *ANAPHYLAXIS, ANGIONEUROTIC EDEMA, HYPERSENSITIVITY REACTIONS.*

DOSAGE: Injection (IV)

Prevention of RSV infections.

Infusion rate of 1.5 mL/kg/hr for 0–15 min. If the clinical condition of the client allows, the rate can be increased to 3.6 mL/kg/hr for the remainder of the infusion. *Do not exceed these rates of infusion.* **Maximum dose/monthly infusion:** 750 mg/kg.

NEED TO KNOW

1. Do not use in clients with selective IgA deficiency who have the potential for developing antibodies to IgA and which could cause anaphylaxis or allergic reactions to blood products that contain IgA.
2. Safety and efficacy have not been determined in children with

congenital heart disease. Give close attention to the infusion rate as side effects may be related to the rate of administration.

3. Antibodies found in immunoglobulin products may interfere with the immune response to live virus vaccines, including those for mumps, rubella, and measles.
4. Enter single-use vial only once. Initiate infusion within 6 hr and complete within 12 hr of removal from the vial.
5. Give separately from other drugs or medications.
6. Give through an IV line using an infusion pump.
7. Assess VS, I&O, and heart/lung/breathing status: prior to infusion, before each rate increase, and thereafter at 30-min intervals until 30 min following infusion completion.
8. Observe for fluid overload (increased HR, increased respiratory rate, crackles, retractions), especially in infants with bronchopulmonary dysplasia. A loop diuretic (e.g., furosemide or bumetanide) should be available for management of fluid overload.
9. The first dose of RSV-IGIV should be given prior to the beginning of the RSV season and monthly throughout the RSV season (in the Northern Hemisphere, from Nov–April) to maintain protection.
10. Report any severe headaches, painful eye movements, drowsiness, fever, N&V, or muscle rigidity (symptoms of aseptic meningitis); must be evaluated to rule out other causes of meningitis.

Salmeterol xinafoate ■ C

(sal-**MET**-er-ole)

Rx: Serevent Diskus.

CLASSIFICATION(S): Sympathomimetic

USES: (1) Long-term (twice daily) maintenance treatment of asthma or in the prevention of bronchospasm in clients 4 years and older with reversible obstructive airway disease. Includes those with symptoms of nocturnal asthma. (2) Prevention of exercise-induced bronchospasm in clients 4 years and older.

ACTION/KINETICS: Selective for beta$_2$-adrenergic receptors located in the bronchi and heart. Acts by stimulating intracellular adenyl cyclase, the enzyme that converts ATP to cyclic AMP. Increased AMP levels cause relaxation of bronchial smooth muscle and inhibition of release of mediators of immediate hypersensitivity, especially from mast cells. **Onset:** Within 20 min. **Duration:** 12 hr. Cleared by hepatic metabolism.

SIDE EFFECTS: Palpitations, tachycardia, tremor, dizziness/vertigo, nervousness, headache, N&V, heartburn, diarrhea, cough, dry/irritated throat, pharyngitis. *PARADOXICAL BRONCHOSPASMS; INCREASED RISK OF SEVERE, FATAL ASTHMA EPISODES; IMMEDIATE HYPERSENSITIVITY REACTIONS.*

DOSAGE: Powder for Inhalation

Bronchospasm, asthma, including nocturnal asthma.

Children, 4 years and over: One inhalation (50 mcg) twice a day (morning and evening, approximately 12 hr apart). If a previously effective dose fails to provide the usual response, seek medical advice immediately as this is often a sign of destabilization of asthma. If symptoms arise in the period between doses, use a short-acting, inhaled beta$_2$-agonist for immediate relief.

Prevention of exercise-induced bronchospasms.

Children, over 4 years: One inhalation (50 mcg) at least 30 min before exercise. Protection may last up to 9 hr in adolescents and up to 12 hr in those 4–11 years. Additional doses should not be used for 12 hr. In those who are receiving salmeterol twice daily, do not use additional salmeterol for prevention of exercise-induced bronchospasm.

NEED TO KNOW

1. Long-acting beta$_2$-adrenergic agonists, such as salmeterol, may increase the risk of asthma-related death. Therefore, when treating clients with asthma, salmeterol should only be

used as additional therapy for clients not adequately controlled on other asthma-controller medications (e.g., low-to medium-dose inhaled corticosteroids) or whose disease severity clearly warrants initiation of treatment with two maintenance therapies, including salmeterol.

2. The safety of more than 8 inhalations per day of short-acting beta$_2$-agonists with salmeterol has not been established.
3. For the inhalation of powder (Diskus), a built-in dose counter shows the number of doses remaining. The inhalation device is not reusable; discard after every blister has been used or 6 weeks after removal from the moisture-protective foil overwrap, whichever comes first.
4. Review proper use (with actuator) and obtain instruction. Shake well. Use the inhalation device in a level, horizontal position. Do not use a spacer.
5. Do not use drug during an acute asthma attack.
6. May experience palpitations, chest pain, headaches, tremors, nervousness, dizziness, drowsiness as side effects. Report immediately if chest pain, fast pounding irregular heartbeat, hives, increased wheezing, or difficulty breathing occurs.

Terbutaline sulfate

(ter-**BYOU**-tah-leen)

Rx: Brethine.

B

CLASSIFICATION(S): Sympathomimetic, direct-acting

USES: Prophylaxis and treatment of bronchospasm in clients 12 years and older with asthma and reversible bronchospasms associated with bronchitis and emphysema.

ACTION/KINETICS: Specific beta-2 receptor stimulant, resulting in bronchodilation and relaxation of peripheral vasculature. Minimum beta-1 activity. **PO, Onset:** 30 min; **maximum effect:** 2–3 hr; **duration:** 4–8 hr. **SC, Onset:** 5–15 min; **maximum effect:** 30

min–1 hr; **duration:** 1.5–4 hr. **Inhalation, Onset:** 5–30 min; **time to peak effect:** 1–2 hr; **duration:** 3–6 hr.
SIDE EFFECTS: Palpitations, tremor, dizziness/vertigo, nervousness/tension, N&V, PVCs/arrhythmias, drowsiness, headache.

DOSAGE: Tablets

Bronchodilation.

Children, over 15 years: 5 mg 3 times per day q 6 hr during waking hours, not to exceed 15 mg q 24 hr. If disturbing side effects are observed, dose can be reduced to 2.5 mg 3 times per day without loss of beneficial effects. Anticipate use of other therapeutic measures if client fails to respond after second dose. **12–15 years:** 2.5 mg 3 times per day, not to exceed 7.5 mg q 24 hr.

NEED TO KNOW

1. Safe use in children less than 12 years not established.
2. Observe respiratory client for evidence of drug tolerance and rebound bronchospasm.
3. Take oral medication with meals to minimize GI upset.
4. Report any persistent or bothersome side effects. Do not increase dose or frequency if symptoms are not relieved. Report so dose can be reevaluated.
5. May use analgesic to relieve headache.
6. Increase fluid intake to help liquefy secretions.

Theophylline

(thee-**OFF**-ih-lin) **C**

Rx: Capsules, Extended-Release or Timed-Release: Slo-Bid Gyrocaps, Theo-24. **Capsules, Immediate-Release:** Bronkodyl, Elixophyllin. **Elixir:** Asmalix, Elixophyllin, Lanophyllin. **Syrup:** Accurbron. **Tablets, Extended-Release or Timed-Release:** T-Phyl, Theochron, Theolair-SR, Theophylline Extended-Release, Theophylline SR, Uniphyl.

CLASSIFICATION(S): Antiasthmatic, xanthine derivative

USES: (1) Prophylaxis and treatment of bronchial asthma. (2) Reversible bronchospasms associated with chronic bronchitis and emphysema.

ACTION/KINETICS: Theophylline stimulates the CNS, directly relaxes the smooth muscles of the bronchi (relieve bronchospasms) and pulmonary blood vessels, produces diuresis, inhibits uterine contractions, stimulates gastric acid secretion, and increases the rate and force of contraction of the heart. Theophyllines may alter the calcium levels of smooth muscle, blocking adenosine receptors, inhibiting the effect of prostaglandins on smooth muscle, and inhibiting the release of slow-reacting substance of anaphylaxis and histamine. Well absorbed PO liquids. **Time to peak serum levels, oral solution:** 1 hr; **extended-release capsules and tablets:** 4–7 hr. **Therapeutic plasma levels:** 10–20 mcg/mL. **$t_{1/2}$:** 1–9 hr in children, 20–30 hr for premature neonates. Because of great variations in the rate of absorption (due to dosage form, food, dose level) as well as its extremely narrow therapeutic range, theophylline therapy is best monitored by determination of the serum levels. Excretion is through the kidneys.

SIDE EFFECTS: N&V, diarrhea, headache, insomnia, irritability. Side effects are uncommon at serum theophylline levels less than 20 mcg/mL.

DOSAGE: Capsules, Immediate-Release; Elixir; Syrup

Bronchodilator, acute attacks, in clients not currently on theophylline.

Children, 1–9 years, PO loading dose: 5 mg/kg; **maintenance:** 4 mg/kg q 6 hr. **9–16 years, PO loading dose:** 5 mg/kg; **maintenance:** 3 mg/kg q 6 hr. **Infants, premature, initial maintenance dose, 24 or less days postnatal:** 1 mg/kg q 12 hr; **more than 24 day postnatal:** 1.5 mg/kg q 12 hr. **Infants, 6–52 weeks, initial maintenance dose:** Calculate as follows:

([0.2 × age in weeks] + 5) × kg = 24 hr dose in mg. For those 26 weeks of age or less, divide into q 8 hr dosing and for those 26–52 weeks of age, divide into q 6 hr dosing. Guide final dosage by serum levels after reaching steady state.

Bronchodilator, acute attacks, in clients currently receiving theophylline.

Children, up to 16 years: If possible, a serum theophylline level should be obtained first. Then, base loading dose on the premise that each 0.5 mg theophylline/kg lean body weight will increase in serum theophylline levels about 1 mcg/mL. If immediate therapy is needed and a serum level cannot be obtained, a single dose of the equivalent of 2.5 mg/kg of anhydrous theophylline in a rapidly absorbed form will raise serum levels by about 5 mcg/mL. If the client is not experiencing theophylline toxicity, this dose is unlikely to result in dangerous side effects.

Chronic therapy, based on anhydrous theophylline.

Children, initial: 16 mg/kg/24 hr, up to a maximum of 400 mg/day in three to four divided doses at 6–8-hr intervals; **then,** dose can be increased in 25% increments at 2–3 day intervals up to a maximum, as follows: **Over 16 years:** 13 mg/kg, not to exceed 900 mg/day; **12–16 years:** 18 mg/kg/day; **9–12 years:** 20 mg/kg/day; **1–9 years:** 24 mg/kg/day.

DOSAGE: Capsules, Extended-Release or Timed-Release; Tablets, Extended-Release or Timed-Release

Bronchodilator, chronic therapy, based on equivalent of anhydrous theophylline.

Children, over 12 years, initial: 4 mg/kg q 8–12 hr; **then,** dose may be increased by 2–3 mg/kg/day at 3-day intervals up to the following maximum doses (without measuring serum levels): **16 years and older:** 13 mg/kg/day or 900 mg/day, whichever is less; **12–16 years:** 18 mg/kg/day.

DOSAGE: Elixir; Syrup

Neonatal apnea.

Loading dose: Using the equivalent of anhydrous theophylline administered by NGT, 5 mg/kg; **maintenance:** 2 mg/kg/day in two to three divided doses given by NGT.

NEED TO KNOW

1. Use with caution in premature infants due to the possible accumulation of caffeine. Xanthines are not usually tolerated by small children because of excessive CNS stimulation.
2. Individualize chronic dosage to maintain serum levels of 10–20 mcg/mL.
3. Calculate dosage based on lean body weight (theophylline does not distribute to body fat). Once stabilized on a dosage, serum levels tend to remain constant.
4. The extended-release tablets or capsules are not recommended for children less than age 6. Dosage for once-a-day products has not been established in children less than 12 years of age.
5. Serum levels may vary significantly following brand interchange.
6. To avoid epigastric pain, take with a snack or with meals. Take ATC and only as prescribed; more is *not* better. Do not crush, dissolve, chew, or break slow-release forms of the drug.
7. May cause dizziness, evaluate drug effects before performing activities that require mental alertness. Report S&S of toxicity

such as N&V, anorexia, insomnia, restlessness/irritability, hyperexcitability; will need drug levels and ECG to assess for arrhythmias.

8. Avoid caffeine- and xanthine-containing beverages and foods (chocolate, coffee, colas) and daily intake of charbroiled foods; increases drug side effects.
9. Hold medication and report side effects or excessive CNS depression/stimulation in children and infants (unable to report side effects).

Ticarcillin disodium and Clavulanate potassium B

(tie-kar-**SILL**-in, klav-you-**LAN**-ate)

Rx: Timentin.

CLASSIFICATION(S): Antibiotic, penicillin

USES: (1) Septicemia, including bacteremia. (2) Lower respiratory tract infections. (3) Bone and joint infections. (4) Skin and skin structure infections. (5) UTIs (complicated and uncomplicated). (6) Peritonitis due to β-lactamase producing strains of *E. coli, K. pneumoniae,* and *Bacteroides fragilis* group.

ACTION/KINETICS: Contains clavulanic acid, which protects the breakdown of ticarcillin by beta-lactamase enzymes, thus ensuring appropriate blood levels of ticarcillin.

SIDE EFFECTS: Hypersensitivity, N&V, gastritis, stomatitis, diarrhea, skin rashes.

DOSAGE: IV Infusion

Mild to moderate infections.

Children, 60 kg or more: 3.1 grams q 6 hr; **less than 60 kg:** 200 mg/kg/day (dosed at 50 mg/kg/dose) q 6 hr.

Severe infections.

Children, 60 kg or more: 3.1 grams q 4 hr; **less than 60 kg:** 300 mg/kg/day (dosed at 50 mg/kg/dose) q 4 hr.

NEED TO KNOW

1. Administer over a 30-min period, either through a Y-type IV infusion or by direct infusion.
2. Continue treatment for at least 2 days after S&S of infection have disappeared. The usual duration is 10–14 days.
3. This product is incompatible with sodium bicarbonate.
4. If used with another anti-infective agent (e.g., an aminoglycoside), give each drug separately.
5. Drug is administered parenterally to treat serious infections.
6. Report any symptoms of bleeding abnormalities, such as small purple spots on skin, easy bruising, or frank bleeding.
7. Extremity swelling, weight gain, or difficulty breathing may be precipitated by drug's large sodium content.

Tolmetin sodium (TOLL-met-in) ■ C

CLASSIFICATION(S): Nonsteroidal anti-inflammatory
USES: Juvenile rheumatoid arthritis.
ACTION/KINETICS: Peak plasma levels: 30–60 min. **$t\frac{1}{2}$:** 2–7 hr. **Therapeutic plasma levels:** 40 mcg/mL. **Onset, anti-inflammatory effect:** Within 1 week; **duration, anti-inflammatory effect:** 1–2 weeks. Inactivated in liver and excreted in urine.
SIDE EFFECTS: Hypertension, headache, dizziness, asthenia/malaise, diarrhea, N&V, flatulence, abdominal/GI distress, peripheral edema, edema.

DOSAGE: Capsules; Tablets

Juvenile rheumatoid arthritis.

Children, 2 years and older, initial: 20 mg/kg/day in 3–4 divided doses to start; **then,** 15–30 mg/kg/day. Doses higher than 30 mg/kg/day are not recommended. Beneficial effects may not be observed for several days to a week.

NEED TO KNOW

1. Safety and efficacy have not been determined in children less than 2 years.
2. Doses should be spaced so that one dose is taken in the morning on arising, one during the day, and one at bedtime.
3. May administer with meals, milk, a full glass of water, or antacids if gastric irritation occurs. Never administer with sodium bicarbonate.
4. Drug may cause drowsiness or dizziness. Report any unusual bruising or bleeding, weight gain, edema, fever, blood in urine, or increased joint pain.

Topiramate

(toh-**PYRE**-ah-mayt)

Rx: Topamax.

C

CLASSIFICATION(S): Anticonvulsant, miscellaneous

USES: (1) Adjunct treatment for partial onset seizures in children, 2–16 years. (2) Adjunct treatment for primary generalized tonic-clonic seizures in children, 2–16 years old. (3) Adjunct treatment of seizures associated with Lennox-Gastaut syndrome in clients 2 years and older. (4) Monotherapy in clients 10 years and older to treat partial-onset or primary generalized tonic-clonic seizures.

ACTION/KINETICS: The following effects may contribute to the anticonvulsant activity. (1) Action potentials seen repetitively by sustained depolarization of neurons are blocked in a time-dependent manner, suggesting an effect to block sodium channels. (2) Increases the frequency at which GABA activates $GABA_A$ receptors, thus enhancing the ability of GABA to cause a flux of chloride ions into neurons (i.e., enhanced effect of the inhibitory transmitter, $GABA_A$). (3) Antagonizes the ability of kainate to activate the kainate/AMPA subtype of excitatory amino acid aspartate, thus reducing the excitatory effect. (4) Inhibits the carbonic anhydrase enzyme, particularly isozymes II and IV. Rapidly absorbed; **peak plasma levels:** About 2 hr. Bioavailability is about 80%. **t½, elimi-**

nation: 21 hr. **Steady state:** About 4 days in those with normal renal function. Excreted mostly unchanged in the urine.
SIDE EFFECTS: Dizziness, paresthesia, ataxia, anxiety, confusion, nervousness, depression, fatigue, somnolence, insomnia, URTI, anorexia, rhinitis, abnormal vision, diplopia, nystagmus, tremor, nausea. *PANCREATITIS, HEPATIC FAILURE (INCLUDING FATALITIES), BRONCHOSPASM, PULMONARY EMBOLISM.*

DOSAGE: Capsules, Sprinkle; Tablets

Epilepsy, monotherapy.

Children, 10 years and older: 400 mg/day in 2 divided doses. Achieve this dosage using the following titration schedule: **Week 1:** 25 mg in the morning and evening; **Week 2:** 50 mg in the morning and evening; **Week 3:** 75 mg in the morning and evening; **Week 4:** 100 mg in the morning and evening; **Week 5:** 150 mg in the morning and evening; **Week 6:** 200 mg in the morning and evening.

Epilepsy, adjunctive therapy: Partial seizures, primary generalized tonic-clonic seizures, Lennox-Gastaut syndrome.

Children, 17 years and older, initial: 25–50 mg/day; then, titrate in increments of 25 to 50 mg/week until an effective daily dose is reached. The recommended total daily dose is 200–400 mg/day; doses greater than 1,600 mg/day have not been studied. **2–16 years:** Begin titration at 25 mg or less (based on a range of 1–3 mg/kg/day) nightly for the first week. Then, increase dose at 1- or 2-week intervals by increments of 1–3 mg/kg/day (given in 2 divided doses) to reach optimal clinical response. The recommended total daily dose is 5–9 mg/kg/day in two divided doses.

NEED TO KNOW

1. Clients taking the drug, especially children, should be monitored for decreased sweating and hyperthermia, especially those exposed to elevated environmental temperatures and/or engaged in vigorous activity.

2. Safety and efficacy have not been determined in children less than 2 years of age for adjunctive therapy of partial onset seizures, primary generalized tonic-clonic seizures, or seizures associated with Lennox-Gastaut syndrome.
3. The sprinkle capsule is bioequivalent to the tablet and thus may be substituted as therapeutically equivalent.
4. If necessary, withdraw topiramate gradually to minimize the risk of increased seizure frequency.
5. Take exactly as prescribed. Due to the bitter taste of the drug, do not break tablets. Can be taken without regard for meals. Do not stop drug abruptly due to risk of increased seizure frequency.
6. For sprinkle capsules, either swallow whole or carefully open capsule and sprinkle the entire contents on a small amount (teaspoon) of soft food. Swallow the drug/food mixture immediately. Do not chew and do not store for future use.
7. Increase fluid intake to decrease substance concentration as drug may precipitate renal stone formation by increasing urinary pH and reducing urinary citrate excretion.

Triamcinolone acetonide ■ C

(try-am-**SIN**-oh-lohn)

Rx: Inhalation Aerosol: Azmacort, Nasacort AQ, Nasacort HFA.

CLASSIFICATION(S): Glucocorticoid

USES: (1) PO inhalation is used for maintenance treatment of chronic asthma (use Azmacort). (2) Intranasal for seasonal and perennial allergic rhinitis in children 6 years and older (use Nasacort AQ or HFA).

ACTION/KINETICS: The anti-inflammatory effect is due to inhibition of prostaglandin synthesis. The drug also inhibits accumulation of macrophages and leukocytes at sites of inflammation and inhibits phagocytosis and lysosomal enzyme release. More potent than prednisone. Intermediate-acting. Has no mineralocorticoid activity. **Onset:** Several hours. **Duration:** One or more weeks. **$t_{1/2}$:** Over 200 min. Metabolized by the liver. About 60% excreted in the feces and 40% in the urine. **$t_{1/2}$, after intranasal use:** 3.1 hr.

SIDE EFFECTS: After nasal/respiratory use: Burning/dryness of nasal passages, nasal/throat irritation, sneezing, epistaxis, cough.

DOSAGE: Aerosol, Oral (Azmacort)

Children, 6–12 years: 1–2 inhalations (100–200 mcg) 3–4 times per day or 2–4 inhalations (200–400 mcg) twice a day, not to exceed 1,200 mcg/day (i.e., 12 inhalations). Use in children less than 6 years has not been determined.

DOSAGE: Intranasal Spray (Nasacort AQ, Nasacort HFA)

Seasonal and perennial allergic rhinitis.

Nasacort AQ: Children, 12 years, initial and maximum dose: 2 sprays (110 mcg) in each nostril once daily (total of 220 mcg once daily). **6–11 years:** 1 spray (55 mcg) in each nostril (total of 110 mcg) once daily; maximum recommended dose is 220 mcg/day as 2 sprays/nostril once daily. Not recommended for children less than 6 years. **Nasacort HFA: Children, 6–11 years:** 220 mcg/day given as 2 sprays (55 mcg/spray) in each nostril once a day. Once maximum effect has been reached, titrate dose to the minimum effective dose. Not recommended for children less than 6 years.

NEED TO KNOW

1. Azmacort Aerosol: Particular care is needed in clients who are transferred from systemically active corticosteroids to triamcinolone inhalation aerosol because deaths due to adrenal insufficiency have occurred in asthmatic clients during and after transfer from systemic corticosteroids to aerosolized steroids in recommended doses.
2. Initially, use aerosol concomitantly with a systemic steroid. After 1 week, initiate a gradual withdrawal of systemic steroid. Make next reduction after 1–2 weeks, depending on response. If symptoms of insufficiency occur, dose of systemic steroid

can be increased temporarily. Also, dose of systemic steroid may need to be increased in times of stress or during a severe asthmatic attack.

3. For Nasacort AQ, individualize to the minimum effective dose to reduce the chance of side effects.
4. Triamcinolone acetonide nasal spray for allergic rhinitis may be effective as soon as 12 hr after initiation of therapy. Reevaluate if improvement is not seen within 2–3 weeks.
5. For best results, store Azmacort canister at room temperature and shake well before use. Do not puncture and do not use or store near heat or open flame; exposure to temperatures greater than 48.8°C (120°F) may cause bursting.
6. Nasacort AQ is viscous at rest but a liquid when shaken. This allows the drug to stay in the nasal airways at the site of inflammation for up to 2 hr.
7. Take at the same time each day. Assess mouth and report any evidence of oral lesions with inhaled therapy.
8. Report evidence of abnormal bruising/bleeding, weight gain, swelling of extremities, or SOB.
9. For Nasacort AQ, prime the nasal spray before use by pushing down on the actuator until a fine spray appears (5 pumps). If the pump has not been used for more than 14 days, the pump must be reprimed with 1 spray. For Nasacort HFA, the canister must be primed with 3 actuations prior to the first use or after 3 days of non-use.

Trimethobenzamide hydrochloride

(try-meth-oh-**BENZ**-ah-myd)

C

Rx: Pediatric Triban, T-Gen, Tebamide, Tigan, Triban, Trimazide.

CLASSIFICATION(S): Antiemetic

USES: Control nausea and vomiting.

ACTION/KINETICS: Related to the antihistamines but with weak antihistaminic properties. Less effective than the phenothiazines

but has fewer side effects. Appears to control vomiting by depressing the CTZ in the medulla. **Onset: PO and IM,** 10–40 min. **Duration:** 3–4 hr after PO and 2–3 hr after IM. 30%–50% of drug excreted unchanged in urine in 48–72 hr.
SIDE EFFECTS: **After PO use:** Blurred vision, depression, diarrhea, dizziness, drowsiness, headache, muscle cramps, disorientation. **After rectal use:** Dizziness, drowsiness, rectal irritation.

DOSAGE: Capsules

Control nausea and vomiting.

Children, 13.6–40.9 kg (30–90 lbs): 100–200 mg 3 or 4 times per day.

NEED TO KNOW

1. Use only as directed.
2. May cause drowsiness and dizziness.
3. Report any unusual or adverse drug effects, lack of response. Attempt to identify triggers that relate to N&V.

Trimethoprim and Sulfamethoxazole

C

(try-**METH**-oh-prim, sul-fah-meh-**THOX**-ah-zohl)

Rx: Bactrim, Bactrim DS, Bactrim IV, Bactrim Pediatric, Cotrim, Cotrim D.S., Cotrim Pediatric, Septra, Septra DS, Sulfatrim.

CLASSIFICATION(S): Antibiotic, combination
USES: **PO, Parenteral:** (1) UTIs due to *Escherichia coli, Klebsiella, Enterobacter, Pseudomonas mirabilis* and *vulgaris,* and *Morganella morganii.* (2) Enteritis due to *Shigella flexneri* or *S. sonnei.* *(3) Pneumocystis carinii* pneumonitis in children. **PO:** (1) Acute otitis media in children due to *Haemophilus influenzae* or *Streptococcus pneumoniae.* (2) Acute exacerbations of chronic bronchitis due to *H. influenzae* or *S. pneumoniae.*

ACTION/KINETICS: Sulfamethoxazole inhibits bacterial synthesis of dihydrofolic acid by competing with para-aminobenzoic acid. Trimethoprim blocks the production of tetrahydrofolic acid by inhibiting the enzyme dihdrofolate reductase. Thus, this combination blocks two consecutive steps in the bacterial biosynthesis of essential nucleic acids and proteins. The combination is rapidly and completely absorbed after PO use. **Peak plasma levels, after PO:** 1–4 hr; **after IV:** 1–1.5 hr. Urine concentrations are considerably higher than serum levels. **Sulfamethoxazole, t½, after PO:** 10–12 hr; 11.3 hr. **Trimethoprim, t½, after PO:** 8–11 hr; **after IV:** 12.8 hr. t½'s are increased significantly in those with severely impaired renal function. Sulfamethoxazole is metabolized to inactive compounds whereas trimethoprim is metabolized only to a small extent. Both are excreted through the kidneys.

SIDE EFFECTS: N&V, anorexia, rash, urticaria. *PANCREATITIS, AGRANULOCYTOSIS, APLASTIC ANEMIA.*

DOSAGE: Double-Strength Tablets; Oral Suspension; Tablets

UTIs, shigellosis, bronchitis, acute otitis media.

Children: Total daily dose of 8 mg/kg trimethoprim and 40 mg/kg sulfamethoxazole divided equally and given q 12 hr for 10–14 days. (*NOTE:* For shigellosis, give pediatric dose for 5 days.)

Prophylaxis of P. carinii *pneumonia.*

Children: 150 mg/m^2 of trimethoprim and 750 mg/m^2 sulfamethoxazole daily in equally divided doses twice a day on 3 consecutive days per week. Do not exceed a total daily dose of 320 mg trimethoprim and 1,600 mg sulfamethoxazole.

Treatment of P. carinii *pneumonia.*

Children: Total daily dose of 15–20 mg/kg trimethoprim and 100 mg/kg sulfamethoxazole divided equally and given q 6 hr for 14–21 days.

DOSAGE: IV

UTIs, shigellosis, acute otitis media.

Children: 8–10 mg/kg/day (based on trimethoprim) in 2–4 divided doses q 6, 8, or 12 hr for up to 14 days for severe UTIs or 5 days for shigellosis.

Treatment of P. carinii *pneumonia.*

Children: 15–20 mg/kg/day (based on trimethoprim) in 3–4 divided doses q 6–8 hr for up to 14 days.

NEED TO KNOW

1. Do not use in infants under 2 months of age.
2. Administer IV infusion over a 60–90 min period.
3. Do not mix the IV infusion with any other drugs or solutions.
4. Assess for megaloblastic anemia; drug inhibits ability to produce folinic acid.
5. Take only as directed. Complete entire prescription and do not share.
6. Report any symptoms of persistent fever, inflammation/swelling of veins/lymph glands, N&V, rash, joint pain/swelling, mental disturbances, or lack of response.
7. May experience dizziness; use caution with activities that require mental alertness.
8. Avoid prolonged sun exposure.

Valproic acid
(val-**PROH**-ick)

Rx: Depacon, Depakene.

Divalproex sodium
(die-val-**PROH**-ex)

Rx: Depakote, Depakote ER.

D

CLASSIFICATION(S): Anticonvulsant, miscellaneous

USES: PO or IV. (1) Alone or in combination with other anticonvulsants for treatment of complex partial seizures in children 10 years and older that occur either in isolation or in association with other types of seizures. (2) Use as sole and adjunctive therapy to treat simple and complex absence seizures (petit mal). (3) As an adjunct in multiple seizure patterns that include absence seizures.

ACTION/KINETICS: May increase brain levels of the neurotransmitter GABA. Other possibilities include acting on postsynaptic receptor sites to mimic or enhance the inhibitory effect of GABA, inhibiting an enzyme that catabolizes GABA, affecting the potassium channel, or directly affecting membrane stability. Absorption is more rapid with the syrup (sodium salt) than capsules. Rapidly dissociates to the valproic ion in the stomach. Rate of absorption of the ion may vary with the formulation (i.e., liquid, solid, or sprinkle), conditions of use (fasting, after food), and the method of administration (i.e., whether sprinkled on food or taken intact). **Peak levels with syrup:** 15 min–2 hr. **Peak serum levels, capsules and syrup:** 1–4 hr (delayed if the drug is taken with food); **peak serum levels, enteric-coated tablet (divalproex sodium):** 3–4 hr. **t½:** 9–16 hr, with the lower time usually seen in clients taking other anticonvulsant drugs (e.g., primidone, phenytoin, phenobarbital, carbamazepine). **t½, children, less than 10 days:** 10–67 hr; **t½, children over 2 months:** 7–13 hr. **Therapeutic serum levels:** 50–100 mcg/mL, although a good correlation has not been established between daily dose, serum level, and therapeutic effect. Metabolized in the liver and inactive metabolites are excreted in the urine; small amounts of valproic acid are excreted in the feces.

SIDE EFFECTS: Asthenia, headache, somnolence, dizziness, tremor, insomnia, amnesia, nervousness, ataxia, N&V, dyspepsia, diarrhea, abdominal pain, anorexia, flu syndrome, infection, nystagmus, diplopia, amblyopia/blurred vision, thrombocytopenia, alopecia. *ACUTE PANCREATITIS, APLASTIC ANEMIA*.

DOSAGE: Capsules; Capsules, Sprinkle; Delayed-Release and Extended-Release Tablets (Divalproex); Syrup (Valproic Acid)

Complex partial seizures, monotherapy.

Children, 10 years and older: 10–15 mg/kg/day for monotherapy. Increase by 5–10 mg/kg/week until seizures are controlled or side effects occur, up to a maximum of 60 mg/kg/day. If a satisfactory response has not been reached, measure plasma levels to determine whether they are in the usually accepted therapeutic range of 50–100 mcg/mL. When converting to monotherapy, initiate at 10–15 mg/kg/day. Increase the dose by 5–10 mg/kg/week to achieve the optimum clinical effect. Concomitant antiepileptic drug dosage can usually be reduced by approximately 25% every 2 weeks. This reduction may be started at initiation of valproic acid therapy or delayed by 1 to 2 weeks if there is a concern that seizures are likely to occur with a reduction. The speed and duration of withdrawal of the concomitant antiepileptic drug can be highly variable; monitor clients closely during this period for increased seizure frequency.

Complex partial seizures, adjunctive therapy.

Children, 10 years and older: Valproic acid may be added to the client's regimen at a dose of 10–15 mg/kg/day. The dose may be increased by 5–10 mg/kg/week to achieve the optimum clinical response. Usually, the optimum response is seen at daily doses less than 60 mg/kg/day. If the total daily dose exceeds 250 mg, give in divided doses.

Simple and complex absence seizures.

Initial: 15 mg/kg/day, increasing at 1-week intervals by 5–10 mg/kg/day until seizures are controlled or side effects occur. Usual recommended dose is 60 mg/kg/day. If the total daily dose exceeds 250 mg, give in divided doses. Therapeutic valproate serum levels for most clients with absence seizures are from 50–100 mcg/mL.

NEED TO KNOW

1. Children less than 2 years are at considerably increased risk of developing fatal hepatotoxicity, especially those on multiple anticonvulsants, those with congenital metabolic disorders, those with severe seizure disorders accompanied by mental retardation, and those with organic brain disease.
2. Safety and efficacy of divalproex sodium have not been determined for treating acute mania in children less than 18 years and for treating migraine in children less than 16 years. Safety and efficacy of divalproex sodium ER tablets for the prophylaxis of migraines in children has not been established; also, safety and efficacy of divalproex sodium ER for the treatment of complex partial seizures, simple and complex absence seizures, and multiple seizure types (that include absence seizures) have not been determined in children less than 10 years.
3. Divide daily dosage if it exceeds 250 mg/day.
4. Do not confuse Depakote ER, an extended-release divalproex sodium, with Depakote delayed-release. The two forms can not be substituted for each other. Depakote still requires dosing q 8–12 hr whereas Depakote ER is given once daily.
5. To minimize GI irritation, initiate at a lower dose, give with food, or use delayed-release (Depakote).
6. To minimize CNS depression, give at bedtime.
7. Do not abruptly discontinue antiepileptic drugs in clients in whom the drug is given to prevent major seizures, due to the strong possibility of precipitating status epilepticus with accompanying hypoxia that are life-threatening.
8. Delayed-release products may reduce irritating GI side effects. Do not chew tablets or capsules; swallow whole to prevent ir-

ritation of mouth and throat. Do not take antacids, dairy products, or carbonated drinks with drug; hastens dissolution.
9. Sprinkle capsules may be swallowed whole or the capsule opened and the contents sprinkled on a small amount (teaspoonful) of applesauce or pudding. Swallow the mixture immediately; do not chew. Do not store for future use.
10. Report any unexplained fever, sore throat, skin rash, tremors, vision problems, yellow skin discoloration, unusual bruising/bleeding; may have liver toxicity. Abdominal pain, N&V, or anorexia can be symptoms of pancreatitis that require prompt medical evaluation.

Vancomycin hydrochloride

(van-koh-**MY**-sin)

Rx: Vancocin, Vancoled.

C (for capsule only, B)

CLASSIFICATION(S): Antibiotic, miscellaneous

USES: **PO:** (1) Antibiotic-induced pseudomembranous colitis due to *Clostridium difficile.* (2) Staphylococcal enterocolitis. (3) Severe or progressive antibiotic-induced diarrhea caused by *C. difficile* that is not responsive to the causative antibiotic being discontinued; also for debilitated clients. **IV:** (1) Severe staphylococcal infections in clients who have not responded to penicillins or cephalosporins, who cannot receive these drugs, or who have resistant infections. Infections include lower respiratory tract infections, bone infections, endocarditis, septicemia, and skin and skin structure infections. (2) Alone or in combination with aminoglycosides to treat endocarditis caused by *Streptococcus viridans* or *S. bovis.* Must combine with an aminoglycoside to treat endocarditis due to *Streptococcus faecalis.* (3) Prophylaxis of bacterial endocarditis in penicillin-allergic clients who have congenital heart disease, or rheumatic or other acquired or valvular heart disease, if such clients are undergoing dental or surgical procedures of the upper respiratory tract. (4) The parenteral dosage form may be given PO to treat pseudomembranous colitis or staphylococcal enterocolitis due to *C. difficile*.

ACTION/KINETICS: Appears to bind to bacterial cell wall, arresting its synthesis and lysing the cytoplasmic membrane by a mechanism that is different from that of penicillins and cephalosporins. May also change the permeability of the cytoplasmic membranes of bacteria, thus inhibiting RNA synthesis. Bactericidal for most organisms and bacteriostatic for enterococci. Poorly absorbed from the GI tract. Diffuses in pleural, pericardial, ascetic, and synovial fluids after parenteral administration. **Peak plasma levels, IV:** 33 mcg/mL 5 min after 0.5 gram dosage. **t½, after PO:** 2–3 hr for children; **t½, after IV:** from 2–3 hr in children to 6–10 hr for newborns. Primarily excreted in urine unchanged. Auditory and renal function tests are indicated before and during therapy.

SIDE EFFECTS: Ototoxicity (including tinnitus), chills, coughing, drowsiness, anorexia, N&V, weakness, sore throat, fever.

DOSAGE: Capsules; Oral Solution

All PO uses.

Children: 40 mg/kg/day in 3–4 divided doses for 7–10 days, not to exceed 2 grams/day. **Neonates:** 10 mg/kg/day in divided doses.

DOSAGE: IV

Severe staphylococcal infections.

Children: 10 mg/kg/6 hr. **Infants and neonates, initial:** 15 mg/kg for one dose; **then,** 10 mg/kg q 12 hr for neonates in the first week of life and q 8 hr thereafter up to 1 month of age.

Prophylaxis of bacterial endocarditis in dental, oral, or upper respiratory tract procedures in penicillin-allergic clients.

Children: 20 mg/kg vancomycin plus 2 mg/kg gentamicin (IV or IM), not to exceed 80 mg, 1 hr before the procedure. May repeat once, 8 hr after the initial dose.

NEED TO KNOW

1. The parenteral form may be administered PO by diluting the

1-gram vial with 20 mL distilled or deionized water (each 5 mL contains about 250 mg vancomycin).
2. Intermittent infusion is the preferred route, but continuous IV drip may be used.
3. Avoid rapid IV administration because this may result in hypotension, nausea, warmth, and generalized tingling. Administer over 1 hr in at least 200 mL of NSS or D5W.
4. Reduce risk of thrombophlebitis by rotating injection sites or adding additional diluent.
5. Avoid extravasation during injections; may cause tissue necrosis.
6. Complete entire course of drug therapy as prescribed otherwise infection may recur.
7. Report any fullness/ringing in ears, adverse effects, worsening of symptoms or lack of response.

Zafirlukast

(zah-**FIR**-loo-kast)

Rx: Accolate.

B

CLASSIFICATION(S): Antiasthmatic

USES: Prophylaxis and chronic treatment of asthma in children 5 years and older.

ACTION/KINETICS: A selective and competitive antagonist of leukotriene receptors D_4 and E_4, which are components of slow-reacting substance of anaphylaxis. It is believed that cysteinyl leukotriene occupation of receptors causes asthma, including airway edema, smooth muscle constriction, and altered cellular activity associated with the inflammatory process. Zafirlukast inhibits bronchoconstriction caused by sulfur dioxide and cold air in clients with asthma. It also attenuates the early- and late-phase reaction in asthmatics caused by inhalation of antigens such as grass, cat dander, ragweed, and mixed antigens. Rapidly absorbed after PO use. **Peak plasma levels:** 3 hr. **$t_{1/2}$, terminal:** About 10 hr.

Extensively metabolized in the liver by CYP2C9, with about 90% excreted in the feces and 10% in the urine.
SIDE EFFECTS: Headache, N&V, diarrhea, abdominal pain, infection, asthenia, dizziness, fever. *HYPERSENSITIVITY REACTIONS.*

DOSAGE: Tablets
Asthma.
Children, 12 years and older: 20 mg 2 times per day. **7–11 years:** 10 mg 2 times per day; even during symptom-free periods.

NEED TO KNOW
1. Do not use to terminate an acute asthma attack, including status asthmaticus.
2. Safety and efficacy have not been determined in children less than 5 years.
3. Take 1 hr before or 2 hr after meals to prevent loss of bioavailability.
4. Take drug regularly during symptom-free periods. Do not increase or decrease dose without approval.
5. Drug is not appropriate for acute episodes of asthma. Continue all other antiasthma agents as prescribed.
6. Avoid triggers (i.e., dust, chemicals, cigarette smoke, pollutants, pets, and perfumes).

Zidovudine (AZT)
(zye-**DOH**-vyou-deen)
Rx: Retrovir.

■ C

CLASSIFICATION(S): Antiviral, nucleoside reverse transcriptase inhibitor
USES: PO: (1) Prevent HIV transmission from pregnant women to their fetuses. (2) HIV-infected children over 3 months of age who have HIV-related symptoms or are asymptomatic with abnormal laboratory values indicating significant immunosuppression.

ACTION/KINETICS: Zidovudine triphosphate competes with thymidine triphosphate (the natural substrate) for incorporation into growing chains of viral DNA by retroviral reverse transcriptase. Once incorporated, zidovudine triphosphate causes premature termination of the growth of the DNA chain. Delays appearance of AIDS symptoms. Rapidly absorbed from the GI tract and is distributed to both plasma and CSF. **Peak serum levels:** 0.1–1.5 hr. **$t_{1/2}$:** Approximately 1 hr. **$t_{1/2}$, clients younger than 3 months of age:** 13 hr. In neonates 14 days of age or less, bioavailability is greater, total body clearance is slower, and half-life was longer than in pediatric clients over 14 days of age. Metabolized rapidly by the liver and excreted through the urine.

SIDE EFFECTS: Headache, malaise, N&V, anorexia, constipation, asthenia, abdominal cramps/pain, arthralgia, chills, dyspepsia, fatigue, insomnia, musculoskeletal pain, myalgia, neuropathy. *HEPATOMEGALY WITH STEATOSIS, PANCREATITIS, SEIZURES, CARDIOMYOPATHY, RHABDOMYOLYSIS, ANAPHYLAXIS, SEIZURES.*

DOSAGE: Capsules; Oral Solution; Syrup; Tablets

Asymptomatic HIV infections.

Children, 6 weeks–12 years, initial: 160 mg/m^2 q 8 hr (480 mg/m^2/day, not to exceed 200 mg q 8 hr).

Prevent transmission of HIV from mothers to their fetuses (after week 14 of pregnancy).

Infant dosing: 2 mg/kg PO q 6 hr beginning within 12 hr after birth and continuing through 6 weeks of age. Infants unable to take the drug PO may be given zidovudine IV at 1.5 mg/kg, infused over 30 min q 6 hr.

NEED TO KNOW

1. Zidovudine is not a cure for HIV; thus, clients may continue to acquire opportunistic infections and other illnesses associated with AIDS-related complex (ARC) or HIV.
2. Do not mix with blood products or protein solutions.
3. Safety and effectiveness of chronic zidovudine therapy are not

known, especially in those with a less advanced form of disease.

4. When used to prevent maternal-fetal transmission of HIV, zidovudine should be initiated in pregnant women between 14 and 24 weeks of gestation; also, IV zidovudine should be given during labor up until the cord is clamped, and newborn infants should receive zidovudine syrup. Infected mothers may not breast feed.
5. Take with or without food q 4 hr around the clock as ordered; sleep must be interrupted to take medication.
6. Report early S&S of anemia, e.g., SOB, weakness, lightheadedness, palpitations, and increased fatigue as well as muscle aches/pain.
7. Report any S&S of superinfections (e.g., furry tongue, mouth lesions, vaginal/rectal itching, rash).
8. Avoid acetaminophen and any other unprescribed drugs that may exacerbate the toxicity of zidovudine.

Zileuton

(zye-**LOO**-ton)
Rx: Zyflo, Zyflo CR.

C

CLASSIFICATION(S): Antiasthmatic, leukotriene receptor antagonist
USES: Prophylaxis and chronic treatment of asthma in children over 12 years.
ACTION/KINETICS: Specific inhibitor of 5-lipoxygenase; thus, inhibits the formation of leukotrienes. Leukotrienes are substances that induce various biological effects including aggregation of neutrophils and monocytes, leukocyte adhesion, increase of neutrophil and eosinophil migration, increased capillary permeability, and contraction of smooth muscle. By inhibiting leukotriene formation, zileuton reduces bronchoconstriction due to cold air challenge in asthmatics. Rapidly absorbed from the GI tract; **peak plasma levels:** 1.7 hr. Food affects the C_{max} of extended-release

tablets but not immediate-release tablets. Metabolized in liver and mainly excreted through the urine. **$t_{1/2}$:** 2.5 hr (immediate-release) and 3.2 hr (extended-release).

SIDE EFFECTS: Immediate-Release: Headache, dyspepsia, nausea, unspecified pain, abdominal pain, asthenia, accidental injury, myalgia. **Delayed-Release:** Sinusitis, pharyngolaryngeal pain, nausea.

DOSAGE: Tablets

Symptomatic treatment of asthma.

Children, over 12 years: 600 mg 4 times per day; **total daily dose:** 2,400 mg.

DOSAGE: Tablets, Extended-Release

Symptomatic relief of asthma.

Children, 12 years and older: 1,200 mg (two 600 mg tablets) twice daily, within 1 hr after morning and evening meals; **total daily dose:** 2,400 mg.

NEED TO KNOW

1. Safety and efficacy have not been determined in children less than 12 years.
2. Do not decrease dose or stop taking any other antiasthmatics when taking zileuton.
3. Take tablets regularly as directed (may take with meals and at bedtime). Tablets may be swallowed whole or split in half for ease of administration.
4. Take the extended-release tablets within 1 hr of morning and evening meals. Do not chew, cut, or crush extended-release tablets. If a dose is missed, take the next dose at the next scheduled time; do not double the dose.
5. Use caution, may cause dizziness; avoid hazardous activities.
6. Drug will not reverse bronchospasm during acute asthma attack.
7. Report immediately if experiencing right upper quadrant pain,

lethargy, itching, jaundice, fatigue, or flu-like symptoms (S&S of liver toxicity).

APPENDIX 1

Calculating Body Surface Area and Body Mass Index

Body Surface Area (BSA) Calculator

Use the following formulas to calculate the body surface area (BSA) for drug administration. These formulas replace the BSA Nomogram.

BSA (metric) = $\sqrt{\text{(ht [cm] x wt [kg])/3600}}$

BSA (English) = $\sqrt{\text{(ht [in] x wt [lb])/3131}}$

Body Mass Index (BMI) Calculator

You may calculate your BMI to assess if you are overweight

1. Multiply your weight in pounds by 703
2. Multiply your height in inches times itself
3. Divide the first number by the second to give your BMI

For example:

You weigh 190 lb and are 5′5″ (65″) tall

1. 190 x 703 = 133,579
2. 65 x 65 = 4,225
3. 133,579 divided by 4,225 = 31.6

Your BMI is 31.6

A BMI under 18.5 indicates that you are underweight

A BMI between 18.5 and 24.9 is considered a healthy weight

If the BMI is between 25 and 29.9 you are moderately overweight

If the BMI is 30 or more you are extremely obese

A precalculated BMI chart is available in most provider offices.

A precalculated BMI chart is available from the National Institutes of Health at: http://www.nhlbi.nih.gov/guidelines/obesity/bmi_tbl.htm

APPENDIX 2

Elements of a Prescription

To safely communicate the exact elements desired on a prescription, the following items should be addressed:

A. The prescriber: Name, address, phone number, and associated practice/specialty.

B. The client: Name, age/birthdate, address, and any allergies of record.

C. The prescription itself: Name of the medication (generic or trade); dosage form and quantity to be dispensed (e.g., number of tablets or capsules, 1 vial, 1 tube, volume of liquid); the strength of the medication (e.g., 125-mg tablets, 250 mg/5 mL, 80 mg/1 mL, 10%); and directions for use (e.g., 1 tablet PO 3 times per day; 2 gtt to each eye 4 times per day; 1 teaspoonful PO q 8 hr for 10 days; apply a thin film to lesions twice a day for 14 days).

D. Other elements: Date prescription is written, signature of the provider, number of refills, provider number: state license number and Drug Enforcement Agency (DEA) number (when applicable), and brand-product-only indication (when applicable).

A typical prescription follows:

A. Julia Bryan, MSN, RN, CPNP
Pediatric Associates
1611 Kirkwood Highway
Wilmington, DE 19805
302-645-8261

Date: July 10, 20XX

B. For: Kathryn Woods, Age 8
27 East Parkway
Lewes, DE 19958
Rx Amoxicillin susp. 250 mg/5 mL
Disp. 150 mL
Sig: 1 teaspoon PO q 8 hr x 10 days

Refills: 0 Provider signature
Provider/State license number

Interpretation of prescription: The above prescription is written by Certified Pediatric Nurse Practitioner Julia Bryan for Kathryn Woods and is for amoxicillin suspension. The concentration desired is 250 mg/5 mL. The directions for taking the medication are 1 teaspoon (i.e., 5 mL) by mouth every 8 hr for 10 days. The prescriber wants 150 mL dispensed and no refills are allowed.

APPENDIX 3

Drug/Food Interactions

A. DRUGS THAT SHOULD BE TAKEN WHILE FASTING

Ampicillin
Digoxin (avoid high fiber cereals and oatmeal)
Fexofenadine
Lansoprazole
Lisinopril
Penicillin
Phenytoin (if GI distress occurs, may take with food; food effect depends on preparation)
Terbutaline sulfate
Trimethoprim

B. DRUGS THAT SHOULD BE TAKEN WITH FOOD

Aspirin
Carbamazepine (erratic absorption)
Doxycyline
Mebendazole
Nitrofurantoin
Oxcarbazepine
Prednisone
Tolmetin

C. CONSTIPATING AGENTS

Antacids
Anticholinergic drugs
Anticonvulsants
Antihistamines
Antiparkinsonian drugs
BP meds (calcium channel blockers)
Clonidine
Corticosteroids
Diuretics
Ganglionic blocking agents
Iron supplements
Laxatives (when abused)

Lithium
MAO Inhibitors
Muscle relaxants
NSAIDs
Octreotide
Opioids
Phenothiazines
Prostaglandin synthesis inhibitors
Tranquilizers
Tricyclic antidepressants

D. DIARRHEAL AGENTS

Adrenergic neuron blockers: reserpine, guanethidine
Antacids (Mg containing) H_2 receptor antagonists (i.e., ranitidine) PPIs (i.e., omeprazole)
Antiarrhythmics (i.e., quinidine)
Antibiotics (especially broad spectrum agents)
Antihypertensives (beta blockers, ACE Inhibitors)
Anti-inflammatory drugs (NSAIDs, colchicine)
Chemotherapy agents
Cholinergic agonists and cholinesterase inhibitors
Glucophage
Metoclopramide
Misoprostol
Osmotic and stimulant laxatives
Theophylline

E. TYRAMINE CONTAINING FOODS

Moderate amounts of tyramine:
Banana peel
Broad beans
Cheese (all except cream cheese and cottage cheese)
Chianti, vermouth
Concentrated yeast extracts/Brewer's yeast
Fermented cabbage products: sauerkraut, kimchee
Fermented soy products: fermented bean curd, soya bean paste, miso soup
Hydrolyzed protein extracts for sauces, soups, gravies

Imitation cheese
Liquid and powdered protein supplements
Meat extracts
Nonalcoholic beers
Prepared meats (sausage, chopped liver, pate, salami, mortadella)
Raspberries
Some non-United States brands of beer
Yeast products

Significant amounts of tyramine:
Avocado
Chocolate
Cream from fresh pasteurized milk
Distilled spirits
Peanuts
Red and white wines, port wines
Soy sauce
Yogurt

F. FOODS CONTAINING GOITROGENS

Asparagus
Broccoli
Brussels sprouts
Cabbage
Cauliflower
Kale
Lettuce
Millet
Mustard
Other leafy green vegetables
Peaches
Peanuts
Peas
Radishes
Rutabaga
Soy beans

Spinach
Strawberries
Turnip greens
Watercress

G. COUMARIN ANTICOAGULANTS AND DIETARY EFFECTS

Consumption of vitamin K-enriched foods may counteract the effects of anticoagulants since the drugs act through antagonism of vitamin K. Advise client on anticoagulants to maintain a steady, consistent intake of vitamin K-containing foods. The drug monograph for warfarin clearly lists these foods. Additionally, certain herbal teas (green tea, buckeye, horse chestnut, Woodruff, tonka beans, melitot) contain natural coumarins that can potentiate the effects of coumadin and should be avoided. Large amounts of avocado also potentiate the drug's effects. Brussels sprouts, broccoli, spinach, kale, turnip greens, and other cruciferous vegetables increase the catabolism of warfarin thereby decreasing its anticoagulant activities. Caffeinated beverages (i.e., cola, coffee, tea, hot chocolate, chocolate milk) can affect therapy. Alcohol intake of more than three drinks per day can affect clotting times. Herbal supplements can also affect bleeding time: Coenzyme Q10 is structurally similar to vitamin K, feverfew, garlic, and ginseng. Avoid herbal medications while on warfarin therapy.

H. GENERAL DRUG CLASS RECOMMENDATIONS

ACE inhibitors: Take captopril and moexipril 1 hr before or 2 hr after meals; food decreases absorption. Avoid high potassium foods as ACE increases K^+.

Analgesic/Antipyretic: Take on an empty stomach as food may slow the absorption.

Antacids: Take 1 hr after or between meals. Avoid dairy foods as the protein in them can increase stomach acid.

Anti-anxiety agents: Caffeine may cause excitability, nervousness, and hyperactivity lessening the anti-anxiety drug effects.

Antibiotics: Penicillin generally should be taken on an empty stomach; may take with food if GI upset occurs. Do not mix with acidic foods: coffee, citrus fruits, and tomatoes; the acid interferes with absorption of penicillin, ampicillin, erythromycin, and cloxacillin.

Anticoagulants: High vitamin K produces blood-clotting substance and may reduce drug effectiveness. Vitamin E greater than 400 IU may prolong clotting time and increase bleeding risk.

Antidepressant drugs: May be taken with or without food.

Antifungals: Avoid taking with dairy products; avoid alcohol.

Antihistamines: Take on an empty stomach to increase effectiveness.

Bronchodilators with theophylline: High-fat meals may increase bioavailability while high-carbohydrate meals may decrease it. Food increases absorption of Theo-24 and Uniphyl which may cause increased N&V, headache, and irritability.

Cephalosporins: Take on an empty stomach 1 hr before or 2 hr after meals. May take with food if GI upset occurs.

Diuretics: Vary in interactions; some cause loss of potassium, calcium, and magnesium. Avoid salty food and natural black licorice as these increase K and Mg losses. Large doses of vitamin D can elevate blood pressure.

H_2 blockers: May take with or without regard to food.

HMG-CoA reductase inhibitors: Take lovastatin with the evening meal to enhance absorption.

Laxatives: Avoid dairy foods as calcium can decrease absorption.

Macrolides: Take on an empty stomach 1 hr before or 2 hr after meals. May take with food for GI upset.

MAO inhibitors: Have many dietary restrictions, so follow dietary guidelines as prescribed. Foods or alcoholic beverages containing tyramine may cause a fatal increase in BP.

Narcotic analgesics: Avoid alcohol as it may increase sedative effects.

Nitroimadazole (metronidazole): Avoid alcohol or food prepared with alcohol for at least three days after finishing the medicine. Alcohol may cause nausea, abdominal cramps, vomiting, headaches, and flushing.

NSAIDs: Take with food or milk to prevent irritation of the stomach.

Quinolones: Take on an empty stomach 1 hr before or 2 hr after meals. May take with food for GI upset but avoid calcium containing foods such as milk, yogurt, vitamins/minerals containing iron, and antacids because they decrease drug concentrations. Caffeine containing products may lead to excitability and nervousness.

Sulfonamides: Take on an empty stomach 1 hr before or 2 hr after meals. May take with food if GI upset occurs.

Tetracyclines: Take on an empty stomach 1 hr before or 2 hr after meals. May take with food but avoid dairy products, antacids, and vitamins containing iron.

INDEX

Boldface = generic drug name